Perry N. Halkitis, PhD
Leo Wilton, PhD
Jack Drescher, MD
Editors

Barebacking: Psychosocial and Public Health Approaches

Barebacking: Psychosocial and Public Health Approaches has been co-published simultaneously as *Journal of Gay & Lesbian Psychotherapy*, Volume 9, Numbers 3/4 2005.

Pre-publication
REVIEWS,
COMMENTARIES,
EVALUATIONS . . .

" A MUST-HAVE, NEEDED VOLUME for anyone working with HIV at-risk populations. . . . A timely book for those working in the HIV/AIDS field, including researchers and counselors. Psychosocial issues are explored, and clinical applications and case studies are discussed. The editors have assembled a collection that represents the wide topography of 'barebacking,' including the history of the term, definitions, and prevelence. Various truths and myths are explored using quantitive and qualitive methods, all with at-risk populations."

William D. Marelich, PhD
Assistant Professor of Psychology
California State University, Fullerton

More pre-publication
REVIEWS, COMMENTARIES, EVALUATIONS . . .

"IN THIS DARK AGE OF POLITIC- ALLY SELECTIVE SCIENCE AND SIMPLEMINDED APPROACHES TO SEX EDUCATION, THIS BOOK COMES AS A WELCOME RELIEF. Barebacking is a complex and increasingly common phenomenon. These studies address important sociological and psychosexual elements that cause men to partake in insafe sex. Internet sex sites, party drugs, AIDS fatigue, need for intimacy, and low self-esteem are only some of the factors that affect the way men negotiate safety during sex with their partners. While most government health agencies cling to a gravely inadequate 'abstinence only' message, these prominent scientists take a good look at issues that make a real difference. Although these studies are geared toward scientists and clinical workers, I HIGHLY RECOMMEND THIS SOBERING AND ENLIGHTENING BOOK TO ANY SEXUALLY ACTIVE INDIVIDUAL."

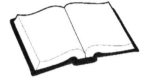

Steven G. Underwood
Author of Gay Men and Anal
Eroticism: Tops, Bottoms, and Versatiles

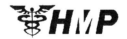

The Haworth Medical Press®
An Imprint of The Haworth Press, Inc.

Barebacking:
Psychosocial and Public
Health Approaches

Barebacking: Psychosocial and Public Health Approaches has been co-published simultaneously as *Journal of Gay & Lesbian Psychotherapy*, Volume 9, Numbers 3/4 2005.

Monographic Separates from the *Journal of Gay & Lesbian Psychotherapy*

For additional information on these and other Haworth Press titles, including descriptions, tables of contents, reviews, and prices, use the QuickSearch catalog at http://www.HaworthPress.com.

Barebacking: Psychosocial and Public Health Approaches, edited by Perry N. Halkitis, PhD, Leo Wilton, PhD, and Jack Drescher, MD (Vol. 9, No. 3/4, 2005). *An examination of the psychological, social, and health issues involving intentional unprotected gay or bisexual sex.*

A Gay Man's Guide to Prostate Cancer, edited by Gerald Perlman, PhD, and Jack Drescher, MD (Vol. 9, No. 1/2, 2005). *"EXCELLENT. . . . HIGHLY RECOMMENDED. Patients reading this book will find themselves here, and professionals will learn what they need to help their patients as they struggle with these emotional topics." (Donald Johannessen, MD, Clinical Assistant Professor of Psychiatry, NYU School of Medicine)*

Handbook of LGBT Issues in Community Mental Health, edited by Ronald E. Hellman, MD, and Jack Drescher, MD (Vol. 8, No. 3/4, 2004). *"COMPREHENSIVE . . . Richly strewn with data, useful addresses of voluntary and other organizations, and case histories." (Michael King, MD, PhD, Professor of Primary Care Psychiatry, Royal Free and University College Medical School, London)*

Transgender Subjectivities: A Clinician's Guide, edited by Ubaldo Leli, MD, and Jack Drescher, MD (Vol. 8, No. 1/2, 2004). *"INDISPENSABLE for diagnosticians and therapists dealing with gender dysphoria, important for researchers, and a direct source of help for all individuals suffering from painful uncertainties regarding their sexual identity." (Otto F. Kernberg, MD, Director, Personality Disorders Institute, Weill Medical College of Cornell University)*

The Mental Health Professions and Homosexuality: International Perspectives, edited by Vittorio Lingiardi, MD, and Jack Drescher, MD (Vol. 7, No. 1/2, 2003). *"PROVIDES A WORLDWIDE PERSPECTIVE that illuminates the psychiatric, psychoanalytic, and mental health professions' understanding and treatment of both lay and professional sexual minorities." (Bob Barrett, PhD, Professor and Counseling Program Coordinator, University of North Carolina at Charlotte)*

Sexual Conversion Therapy: Ethical, Clinical, and Research Perspectives, edited by Ariel Shidlo, PhD, Michael Schroeder, PsyD, and Jack Drescher, MD (Vol. 5, No. 3/4, 2001). *"THIS IS AN IMPORTANT BOOK. . . . AN INVALUABLE RESOURCES FOR MENTAL HEALTH PROVIDERS AND POLICYMAKERS. This book gives voice to those men and women who have experienced painful, degrading, and unsuccessful conversion therapy and survived. The ethics and misuses of conversion therapy practice are well documented, as are the harmful effects." (Joyce Hunter, DSW, Research Scientist, HIV Center for Clinical & Behavioral Studies, New York State Psychiatric Institute/Columbia University, New York City)*

Gay and Lesbian Parenting, edited by Deborah F. Glazer, PhD, and Jack Drescher, MD (Vol. 4, No. 3/4, 2001). *Richly textured, probing. These papers accomplish a rare feat: they explore in a candid, psychologically sophisticated, yet highly readable fashion how parenthood impacts lesbian and gay identity and how these identities affect the experience of parenting. Wonderfully informative. (Martin Stephen Frommer, PhD, Faculty/Supervisor, The Institute for Contemporary Psychotherapy, New York City).*

Addictions in the Gay and Lesbian Community, edited by Jeffrey R. Guss, MD, and Jack Drescher, MD (Vol. 3, No. 3/4, 2000). *Explores the unique clinical considerations involved in addiction treatment for gay men and lesbians, groups that reportedly use and abuse alcohol and substances at higher rates than the general population.*

Barebacking: Psychosocial and Public Health Approaches

Perry N. Halkitis, PhD
Leo Wilton, PhD
Jack Drescher, MD
Editors

Barebacking: Psychosocial and Public Health Approaches has been co-published simultaneously as *Journal of Gay & Lesbian Psychotherapy*, Volume 9, Numbers 3/4 2005.

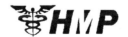

The Haworth Medical Press®
Harrington Park Press®
Imprints of The Haworth Press, Inc.

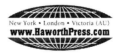

New York • London • Victoria (AU)
www.HaworthPress.com

Published by

The Haworth Medical Press®, 10 Alice Street, Binghamton, NY 13901 1580 USA

The Haworth Medical Press® is an imprint of The Haworth Press, Inc., 10 Alice Street, Binghamton, NY 13904-1580 USA.

Barebacking: Psychosocial and Public Health Approaches has been co-published simultaneously as *Journal of Gay & Lesbian Psychotherapy*, Volume 9, Numbers 3/4 2005.

The development, preparation, and publication of this work has been undertaken with great care. However, the publisher, employees, editors, and agents of The Haworth Press and all imprints of The Haworth Press, Inc., including The Haworth Medical Press® and Pharmaceutical Products Press®, are not responsible for any errors contained herein or for consequences that may ensue from use of materials or information contained in this work. Opinions expressed by the author(s) are not necessarily those of The Haworth Press, Inc. With regard to case studies, identities and circumstances of individuals discussed herein have been changed to protect confidentiality. Any resemblance to actual persons, living or dead, is entirely coincidental.

Cover design by Marylouise E. Doyle

Library of Congress Cataloging-in-Publication Data

Barebacking: psychosocial and public health approaches / Perry N. Halkitis, Leo Wilton, Jack Drescher, editors.
    p. ; cm.
    "Co-published simultaneously as Journal of gay & lesbian psychotherapy, Volume 9, Number 3/4, 2005"
    Includes bibliographical references and index.
    ISBN-10: 0-7890-2173-0 (hard cover : alk. paper)
    ISBN-10: 0-7890-2174-9 (soft cover : alk. paper)
    ISBN-13: 978-0-7890-2173-1 (hard cover : alk. paper)
    ISBN-13: 978-0-7890-2174-8 (soft cover : alk. paper)
    1. AIDS(Disease)–Risk factors. 2. HIV Infections–Risk factors. 3. Gay men–Sexual behavior. 4. Bisexual men–Sexual behavior. 5. Gay men–Psychology. 6. Bisexual men–Psychology. 7. Safe sex in AIDS prevention. 8. Anal sex–Health aspects. 9. Homosexuality, Male–Psychological aspects. 10. Risk-taking (Psychology) I. Halkitis, Perry N. II. Wilton, Leo. III. Drescher, Jack, 1951– IV. Journal of gay & lesbian psychotherapy.
    [DNLM: 1. Homosexuality, Male–psychology. 2. Sexual behavior–psychology. 3. HIV Infections–transmission. 4. Risk Taking. 5. Sexual Partners–psychology.]
RA643.8.B365 2005
362.196'9792–dc22
                                      2004030492

Indexing, Abstracting & Website/Internet Coverage

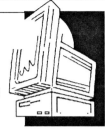

This section provides you with a list of major indexing & abstracting services and other tools for bibliographic access. That is to say, each service began covering this periodical during the year noted in the right column. Most Websites which are listed below have indicated that they will either post, disseminate, compile, archive, cite or alert their own Website users with research-based content from this work. (This list is as current as the copyright date of this publication.)

Abstracting, Website/Indexing Coverage . . . . Year When Coverage Began

- *Abstracts in Anthropology* 1991
- *Academic Index (on-line)* 1992
- *Academic Search Elite (EBSCO)* 1998
- *Academic Search Premier (EBSCO)* 2001
- *British Journal of Psychotherapy* 2005
- *Business Source Corporate: coverage of nearly 3,350 quality magazines and journals; designed to meet the diverse information needs of corporations; EBSCO Publishing <http://www.epnet.com/corporate/bsourcecorp.asp>* 1998
- *Contemporary Women's Issues* 1998
- *EBSCOhost Electronic Journals Service (EJS) <http://ejournals.ebsco.com>* 2004
- *e-psyche, LLC <http://www.e-psyche.net>* 2001
- *Expanded Academic ASAP <http://www.galegroup.com>* 1993
- *Expanded Academic ASAP–International <http://www.galegroup.com>* 1993
- *Expanded Academic Index* 1995
- *Family Index Database <http://www.familyscholar.com>* 2003
- *Family Violence & Sexual Assault Bulletin* 1992
- *GenderWatch <http://www.slinfo.com>* 1999

(continued)

(continued)

*Special Bibliographic Notes related to special journal issues
(separates) and indexing/abstracting:*

- indexing/abstracting services in this list will also cover material in any "separate" that is co-published simultaneously with Haworth's special thematic journal issue or DocuSerial. Indexing/abstracting usually covers material at the article/chapter level.
- monographic co-editions are intended for either non-subscribers or libraries which intend to purchase a second copy for their circulating collections.
- monographic co-editions are reported to all jobbers/wholesalers/approval plans. The source journal is listed as the "series" to assist the prevention of duplicate purchasing in the same manner utilized for books-in-series.
- to facilitate user/access services all indexing/abstracting services are encouraged to utilize the co-indexing entry note indicated at the bottom of the first page of each article/chapter/contribution.
- this is intended to assist a library user of any reference tool (whether print, electronic, online, or CD-ROM) to locate the monographic version if the library has purchased this version but not a subscription to the source journal.
- individual articles/chapters in any Haworth publication are also available through the Haworth Document Delivery Service (HDDS).

Barebacking: Psychosocial and Public Health Approaches

CONTENTS

ABOUT THE EDITORS

Perry N. Halkitis, PhD, is a health and educational psychologist and research methodologist who is Associate Professor and Chair of Applied Psychology at New York University, Director of the Center for Health, Identity, Behavior, and Prevention Studies (CHIBPS, formerly CHEST-NYU), and a research affiliate of the New York University Medical School Center for AIDS Research (CFAR). Dr. Halkitis has worked in the field of HIV/AIDS conducting behavioral research since 1995. His work, which has been funded by the National Institutes of Health, Centers for Disease Control & Prevention, New York City Department of Health, Substance Abuse & Mental Health Services Administration, as well as private organizations, has focused on prevention for HIV-positive people, HIV treatment and adherence issues, methamphetamine and other club drug use in the gay community, bareback behavior and identity, conceptions of masculinity among gay men, genetic resistance to HIV, and spirituality in the LGBT population. Recipient of the 1999 American Psychological Foundation Placek Award, Dr. Halkitis is also the NYU 1999 Daniel E. Griffith's Research Award winner, the 2002 American Psychological Association Emerging Leader for his contributions to the field of HIV/AIDS, the 2002 American Psychological Association Award recipient for Distinguished Contribution to Research in the LGBT Community, and the 2005 HIV Prevention Leader Award from TheBody.com. Dr. Halkitis received his doctorate in Educational Psychology with a specialization in quantitative methods from the Graduate Center, City University of New York.

Leo Wilton PhD, is Assistant Professor in the Departments of Human Development and Africana Studies at Binghamton University, State University of New York. Dr. Wilton specializes in the areas of health psychology; Black psychological development and mental health; multicultural psychology; and lesbian, gay, bisexual, and transgender psychological issues. His scholarly research in the area of primary and secondary HIV prevention has focused on the impact of sociocultural factors as related to sexual/drug-risk behavior and mental health for gay men of color. Dr. Wilton completed his doctoral studies in counseling psychology at New York University (NYU) and a predoctoral clinical psychology fellowship at the Yale University School of Medicine. He completed a three-year postdoctoral research fellowship, competitively funded by the National Institute of Drug Abuse (NIDA), at the Center for HIV/AIDS Educational Studies and Training (CHEST) at NYU. Dr. Wilton has held faculty positions in the Department of Clinical and Counseling Psychology at Teachers College, Columbia University and Department of Applied Psychology at New York University.

Jack Drescher, MD, is a Fellow, Training and Supervising Analyst at the William Alanson White Psychoanalytic Institute. He is Past President of the New York County District Branch, American Psychiatric Association and Chair of the Committee on GLB Concerns of the APA. Author of *Psychoanalytic Therapy and the Gay Man* (1998, The Analytic Press), and Editor-in-Chief of the *Journal of Gay & Lesbian Psychotherapy*, Dr. Drescher is in private practice in New York City.

Preface:
Psychosocial and Public Health
Approaches to Barebacking

The history of Europe is punctuated by long-term wars so costly in terms of human life that people now living question how it was possible for those caught up in these conflicts to maintain some semblance of a normal life or even to survive. Unfortunately, such disruptions are not restricted to the distant past and can even be said to exist within certain communities within our own urban centers. One such community is that of urban gay men, whose experience of the AIDS epidemic can probably best be described by using the metaphor of wartime losses. The way that gay male communities cope with the repercussions of the AIDS epidemic as they enter the third decade of the epidemic will undoubtedly have an enormous influence on how the epidemic continues to evolve within America's largest cities.

As has been so often observed over these long decades, prevention remains our best defense in the fight against AIDS. Less remarked upon has been the prevailing ideologies upon which this fight has been based. One approach to AIDS prevention has been centered on understanding and disrupting the dynamics of viral spread through human populations. This approach has emphasized (1) strict adherence over long periods of time to abstinence and/or condom use in non-monogamous relationships; (2) mutual monogamy within seroconcordant relationships; (3) abstinence from injection drug use and/or no sharing of needles or other drug injection paraphernalia; and (4) treatment of other STIs and HIV infection itself. Many of these elements were prominent in the initial response to the epidemic within gay male communities. One label for this approach is "virus-centered prevention."

[Haworth co-indexing entry note]: "Preface: Psychosocial and Public Health Approaches to Barebacking." Stall, Ronald. Co-published simultaneously in *Journal of Gay & Lesbian Psychotherapy* (The Haworth Medical Press, an imprint of The Haworth Press, Inc.) Vol. 9, No. 3/4, 2005, pp. xxi-xxiii; and: *Barebacking: Psychosocial and Public Health Approaches* (ed: Perry N. Halkitis, Leo Wilton, and Jack Drescher) The Haworth Medical Press, an imprint of The Haworth Press, Inc., 2005, pp. xiii-xv. Single or multiple copies of this article are available for a fee from The Haworth Document Delivery Service [1-800-HAWORTH, 9:00 a.m. - 5:00 p.m. (EST). E-mail address: docdelivery@haworthpress.com].

Available online at http://www.haworthpress.com/web/JGLP
xiii

Another approach the long-term threat of AIDS is one that is more concerned with sustaining a full life, even in the context of a dangerous epidemic. Such approaches are more interested in ensuring that life goals for happiness and fulfilling relationships are met, even when meeting such goals involves increased risk for transmitting HIV infection. It may be that as years of fighting AIDS continue to pass that a greater range of culturally-defined adaptations to the epidemic will develop, among them some that would not be recommended by adherents of virus-centered AIDS prevention efforts.

Certainly the arrival of barebacking on the urban gay male scene suggests that some responses to the epidemic will emerge that are inconsistent with the goal of absolute sexual safety among gay men. This trend raises a question of great importance to prevention work among gay men: what is the best prevention response for individuals who do not manage their sexual lives so that risk of HIV transmission is minimized to the greatest extent possible?

The first step in answering this question would be to understand more about the sexual strategies of barebackers. This is a primary focus, in one way or another, of each of the chapters in this special issue of the *Journal of Gay & Lesbian Psychotherapy*. In addition to this agenda, one might suggest three other possible responses to the barebacking phenomena: (1) to provide rigorous epidemiological data to measure the actual risks of HIV transmission of this behavioral complex; (2) to study new approaches to HIV prevention that might lower the prevalence of very high risk sex among gay men; and (3) to improve treatment and prevention technologies so that risk of transmission even during unprotected anal sex between discordant partners is minimized. The balance of this Preface will address each of these responses in turn.

Although it is a truism that knowledge alone is not sufficient to change behavior, knowledge is generally necessary to support long-term behavioral change. However, it is notable that when it comes to the actual levels of risk for many of the sexual strategies that are described as prominent among barebackers, the epidemiological data are very weak. That is, it remains unclear what the actual level of risks for new HIV transmission are for unprotected anal sex between seropositive partners (i.e., superinfection), for positional strategies (i.e., negative men serving as insertive partners during unprotected anal intercourse with a positive partner) or even the risks association with negotiated safety among non-monogamous male partners (i.e., restricting unprotected anal sex to a primary seroconcordant partnership). Providing affected gay male populations with rigorous epidemiological estimates of the risk for HIV transmission associated with these behaviors may well support their efforts men to reduce their levels of sexual risk. If told that data to measure the actual risk of specific sexual strategies do not exist or are very weak, their motivation to change behaviors might also be at a corresponding weak level.

A second agenda to would be to study new approaches to HIV prevention that might lower the prevalence of very high risk sex among gay men. This topic is addressed in this special issue by Jeffrey Parson's paper on motivational interviewing. Continued research with high-risk men to understand motivations for barebacking (a topic addressed by Richard Wolitski's paper) is certainly indicated. Such work may produce prevention models that address other health challenges faced by high-risk men, such as substance abuse, depression or coping with the cumulative effects of the AIDS epidemic itself. Interventions in these latter areas may lower rates of risk in this population, not to mention the direct positive effects of addressing these important health issues among gay men.

Finally, some responses to the barebacking phenomena might also be biomedical in nature. Increased treatment efficacy for HIV infection, the production of safe and acceptable microbicides and even the development of an AIDS vaccine could reduce the level of risk of HIV transmission associated with barebacking. Each of these agendas is being pursued for their intrinsic value, but may take on additional value as prevention responses to the risks associated with barebacking.

In closing, while the topic of this special issue is barebacking, the central question posed by the study of this phenomena addresses questions that are essential to good public health practice. These include: How can risk reductions be effectively promoted on a population-wide basis for long periods of time? What should the public health response be to community-based responses to dangerous epidemics when the latter run counter to prevailing wisdom? What should the public health response be when individuals choose not to reduce risk after exposure to risk reduction campaigns? What is the proper balance between individual rights and protection of the public health? We all look forward to how continued study of the barebacking phenomena will generate insights relating to these core public health issues.

Ronald Stall, PhD
Chief
Prevention Research Branch
Divisions of HIV/AIDS Prevention
Centers for Disease Control and Prevention
1600 Clifton Road, NE
(M/S E-37)
Atlanta, GA 30309

Introduction:
Why Barebacking?

Perry N. Halkitis, PhD
Leo Wilton, PhD
Jack Drescher, MD

In the late 1970s, a deadly virus which could be transmitted via sex appeared in the midst of an unsuspecting, sexually active community. Before anyone was even aware of the virus' existence, thousands had become infected. By the beginning of the 1980s, gay men in American cities were suddenly afflicted with Kaposi's sarcoma, a rare form of skin cancer more commonly found in equatorial Africa. Unusual, opportunistic infections, indicating some form of immunosuppression, took down young men in their prime. People were dying and although the modes of transmission suggested a biological vector, no specific etiological agent for this "Gay Related Immunodeficiency" would be found for several years. Whatever was causing it, however, appeared to have infiltrated the blood supply, affecting not only hemophiliacs, but potentially endangering anyone who needed a transfusion. There was growing panic and serious public discussion of quarantining gay people–or at least of tattooing them with the modern scarlet letters of what would eventually come to be known as AIDS (Shilts, 1987; Rotello, 1997).

At the time this is being written, it is almost 25 years since AIDS appeared on the American scene as a growing public health concern.

[Haworth co-indexing entry note]: "Introduction: Why Barebacking?" Halkitis, Perry N., Leo Wilton, and Jack Drescher. Co-published simultaneously in *Journal of Gay & Lesbian Psychotherapy* (The Haworth Medical Press, an imprint of The Haworth Press, Inc.) Vol. 9, No. 3/4, 2005, pp. 1-8; and: *Barebacking: Psychosocial and Public Health Approaches* (ed: Perry N. Halkitis, Leo Wilton, and Jack Drescher) The Haworth Medical Press, an imprint of The Haworth Press, Inc., 2005, pp. 1-8. Single or multiple copies of this article are available for a fee from The Haworth Document Delivery Service [1-800-HAWORTH, 9:00 a.m. - 5:00 p.m. (EST). E-mail address: docdelivery@haworthpress.com].

Available online at: http://www.haworthpress.com/web/JGLP
doi:10.1300/J236v09n03_01

Much has happened since then, both bad and good. There has been a terrible loss of life. However, effective means of diagnosing, treating and preventing the spread of AIDS have been found. Yet the number of people infected with HIV continues to grow, despite the development and implementation of numerous educational and psychoeducational efforts.

Public health models often operate under the assumption that unsafe sexual practices are the result of ignorance or lack of knowledge. However, to the amazement and chagrin of those familiar with the epidemic's history, some individuals continue to risk exposing themselves to HIV infection–even when they know how to avoid doing so. Which brings us to the subject of this special issue of the *Journal of Gay & Lesbian Psychotherapy* on barebacking.

Barebacking, which many in the gay community would commonly define as intentional unprotected anal intercourse, was a subject of discussion in the popular press long before academics and clinicians took notice. As early as 1996, Jesse Green wrote of the phenomenon, calling it "Flirting with Suicide," in *The New York Times Magazine*. Then, in 1997, Stephen Gendin wrote of his desire for unprotected anal intercourse (UAI) in a *Poz* magazine entitled "Riding Bareback." He expressed the beliefs and desires of HIV-positive men like himself who felt there was no reason to avoid UAI, as there was no longer any "logical" medical concern about sharing ejaculate with others of the same serostatus. As the phenomenon grew, it was suggested that barebacking was a mechanism by which HIV-positive men could feel closer and more emotionally intimate with their sexual partners (Halkitis, 2001), particularly within a society that continued to stigmatize them for having HIV.

What followed was a growing public discussion about barebacking. Leading gay publications like *The Advocate* (April 13, 1999) and *Poz* (February, 1999) featured cover stories on the subject, offering harm reduction strategies for those engaging in the behavior. In the meantime, debate began to emerge about the health of the gay community in light of this phenomenon. Leading HIV prevention agencies took note, but dismissed the barebacking phenomenon as one confined to only a small subset of men. However, some researchers believed that barebacking behavior was more pervasive than HIV prevention agencies would acknowledge (Halkitis and Parsons, 1998).

While barebacking appears to have begun as a phenomenon confined to those who had already seroconverted, it quickly drew the attention of those who had not. Internet sites dedicated to "raw sex" began to appear.

Today, sites like *barebackcity.com* or *barebacksex.com* provide a venue for barebackers to meet each other. At any given moment, thousands of men, regardless of age, race, or HIV serostatus, log on to these sites in search of sexual partners. Simultaneously within large gay communities, bareback sex parties have grown in popularity. Such events, confined either to one serostatus or open to all (colloquially referred to as "Russian Roulette" parties), permit men to bareback with numerous partners within a brief period of time. In this regard, research has confirmed that barebacking is a phenomenon that cuts across demographics and serostatus (Halkitis and Parsons, 2003; Halkitis, Parsons and Wilton, 2003; Mansergh et al., 2002).

These behaviors are, of course, a matter of great concern. The rate of new HIV diagnoses among men having sex with men (MSM) has increased by 14% between 1999 and 2001 (Valdiserri, 2003). High rates of infection have been noted among young MSM, especially those of color (Koblin et al., 2000; Valleroy et al., 2000). There have been dramatic increases in the incidence of sexually transmitted infections (STIs), other than HIV, such as gonorrhea (Centers for Disease Control and Prevention, CDC, 1999; 2000) and syphilis (Ciesielski, 2003). This trend has become so alarming that the CDC released a public health alert focused on taking action to combat increases in STIs and HIV infection in this population (CDC, 2001). Wolitski et al. (2001) warned that these unsafe behaviors might lead to a resurgence in the HIV epidemic in the MSM community. Sadly, some research now appears to suggest that this is, in fact, happening (Valdiserri, 2003).

While no evidence currently points to a direct link between barebacking and a rise in HIV infections, these epidemiological trends coincide with the growing popularity of barebacking within the gay community. It should be noted that this rise in infections also parallels increases in the use of club drugs, reliance on the Internet as a source of sexual connection in the gay community, implementation of Highly Active Antiretroviral Therapy to fight AIDS, and decreased funding for HIV prevention in the United States. Thus, multiple factors are likely at play. Nevertheless, epidemiological data suggest that unsafe sex is escalating in the gay male communities of the United States, and occurring within a cultural and sociological context very different from one that existed 10 years ago.

It has been suggested that barebacking represents a very different type of sexual experience than those traditionally examined in HIV behavioral research, and that the construct of barebacking is poorly defined (Halkitis et al., 2005) . Further, MSM may use differing heuristics in making sense of barebacking, and in negotiating the sexual safety associated with it. Even among the published studies above, the behavioral research regarding barebacking falls short in two main domains: (1) there may be incongruity between "professional" definitions of barebacking and the manner in which the behavior is understood at the community-level; and (2) there is no understanding of why some men develop along trajectories that may lead to barebacking behaviors while others do not. Further, there is no understanding of the transition points that place men at risk, or the risk or protective bases which predispose men to behave in certain sexual manners. What most researchers can agree upon is that barebacking refers to sex without a condom, and most probably to "intentional" anal sex without a condom (Goodroad et al., 2000). How an individual's intentions for unsafe anal sex or other factors related to this behavior remains unclear. With that in mind, some (Halkitis et al., 2004) have proposed differentiating between barebacking behavior and a "barebacking identity." In other words, a man who thinks of himself as a "barebacker" does not necessarily have the same psychological profile or motivations as another who eschews a "barebacking identity" but who nevertheless practices unprotected anal sex.

Regardless of whether one has a bareback identity or not, the practice of UAI has immediate consequences for the health of the gay community. For HIV-negative men, initial infection with HIV and infections with other STIs is the most immediate consequence of unsafe transmission behaviors. There is also a potential for initial infection with medication resistant/untreatable HIV mutant variants (Boden et al., 1999). For HIV-positive gay and bisexual men, unsafe sexual acts may place them at risk for "superinfection" (Jost et al., 2002), rapid loss of CD4 cells (Wiley et al., 2000), and risk for contracting other STIs which may lead to immune system deterioration (Bonell, Weatherburn and Hickson, 2000). Clearly these are matters of great concern that require our attention.

An earlier issue of the *JGLP* explored barebacking from the perspective of psychodynamically-oriented clinicians (Blechner, 2002; Cheuvront, 2002; Drescher, 2002; Forstein, 2002; Orange, 2002). With this volume, we explore the barebacking phenomenon further, considering the ideas of those working in the field as well as those who can provide both research and clinical perspectives on the topic. While every question will not be answered, a deeper understanding of barebacking may be achieved by considering a range of sociological, psycho-behavioral, and clinical perspectives. The aim is to provide clinicians working with this population of gay men some insights into these unsafe sexual behaviors, as well as to raise questions for themselves, their patients and for researchers seeking to make sense of this phenomenon.

We begin with Richard J. Wolitski, PhD's "The Emergence of Barebacking Among Gay and Bisexual Men in the United States: A Public Health Perspective," in which he considers the reasons for the emergence of barebacking. Wolitski examines the roles of HIV treatment advances, HIV fatigue, the Internet, drug abuse, changes in HIV prevention programs, and safer-sex decision making in helping to explain the rise of the barebacking phenomenon, and offers suggestions for future research in this domain.

In "What's in a Term? How Gay and Bisexual Men Understand Barebacking," Perry N. Halkitis, PhD, Leo Wilton, PhD and Paul Galatowitsch, PhD provide an overview of how gay and bisexual men understand barebacking through an empirical study of the population. Their work suggests that the construct is not uniformly understood by gay and bisexual men, and indicates that one of the challenges for prevention efforts rests with the differences in conceptual understanding of what barebacking actually is or means to gay and bisexual men.

The role of race, culture, and drug abuse–and the synergy of these factors with regard to barebacking–is explored in Leo Wilton, PhD, Perry N. Halkitis, PhD, Gary English, and Michael Roberson's "An Exploratory Study of Barebacking, Club Drug Use, and Meanings of Sex in Black and Latino Gay and Bisexual Men in the Age of AIDS." Using both quantitative and qualitative methods, the authors demonstrate that barebacking behavior may vary along lines of race and may be differentially affecting the drug use in which men are engaging.

Two articles follow in which the role of the Internet is examined empirically. The first is "Evidence of HIV Transmission Risk in Barebacking Men-Who-Have-Sex-With-Men: Cases from the Internet," by Alvin G. Dawson, Jr., MA, Michael W. Ross, PhD, Doug Henry, PhD and Anne Freeman, MSPH. Their work indicates that the Internet provides a venue by which men who seek bareback sex may identify potential partners. However, many of those who advertise on the Internet partake in "sero-sorting, a harm reduction strategy to reduce HIV transmission by selecting sexual partners based on serostatus. Their findings are corroborated by David S. Bimbi, MA and Jeffrey T. Parsons, PhD in "Barebacking Among Internet Based Male Sex Workers." Theirs is a study of harm reduction strategies utilized by sex workers with their sexual partners.

In "Attitudes Toward Unprotected Anal Intercourse: Assessing HIV-Negative Gay or Bisexual Men," Ariel Shidlo, PhD, Huso Yi, PhD and Boaz Dalit, PsyD provide a measurement tool for assessing unprotected anal intercourses among gay and bisexual men that can be used by clinicians and clients in understanding the elements that may predispose men to engage in risky sexual behavior and place themselves at risk for HIV seroconversion. The authors also provide guidance for counseling men who may be at risk.

This volume concludes with two clinical perspectives on barebacking. First is "Motivating the Unmotivated: A Treatment Model for Barebackers," in which Jeffrey T. Parsons, PhD provides an overview of Motivational Interviewing. He illustrates how such an approach to therapeutic intervention may be applied to addressing barebacking behavior with clients. In "Condomless Sex: Considerations for Psychotherapy with Individual Gay Men and Male Couples Having Unsafe Sex," Michael Shernoff, MSW, provides a first-hand account of his experiences in treating both single and coupled men who may be engaging in bareback behavior.

While the focus of this volume is on the gay male population, the practice of unsafe sex is not confined solely to the latter and high risk sexual behavior has been documented across subgroups of the HIV-positive population (Burman et al., 2004). Recent data indicate the rise of HIV infections in the heterosexual population as well. In fact, infections among women in the United States through heterosexual contact have steadily increased in the last several years (Whitmore et al., 2004). Obviously, additional public health strategies need to be aware of how individuals consider and make sense of HIV in their lives.

Perry N. Halkitis, PhD
Leo Wilton, PhD
Jack Drescher, MD

REFERENCES

Blechner, M.J. (2002), Intimacy, pleasure, risk and safety: Commentary on Cheuvront's "High-risk sexual behavior in the treatment of HIV-negative patients." *J. Gay & Lesbian Psychotherapy*, 6(3):27-34.

Boden, D., Hurley, A., Zhang, L., Cao, Y., Jones, E., Tsay, J., Farthing, C., Limoli, K., Parkin, N., & Markowitz, M. (1999), HIV-1 drug resistance in newly infected individuals. *JAMA*, 282(1):135-141.

Bonnel, C., Weatherburn, P., & Hickson, F. (2000), Sexually transmitted infection as a risk factor for homosexual HIV transmission: A systematic review of epidemiological studies. *International J. STD & AIDS*, 11:697-700.

Burman, W., Neuhaus, J., Reitmeijer, C., Douglas, J., & McCartin (2004), *HIV Transmission Risk Among Patients Enrolled in a Large Clinical Trial Evaluating Treatment Interruption.* Paper presented at the XV International Aids Conference, Bangkok, Thailand, July.

Centers for Disease Control & Prevention (1999), Increases in unsafe sex and rectal gonorrhea among men who have sex with men–San Francisco, California, 1994-1997. *Morbidity & Mortality Report*, January 29, 48(3):45-58.

Centers for Disease Control and Prevention (CDC) (October 30-31, 2000), Consultation on recent trends in STD and HIV morbidity and risk behaviors among MSM. Meeting Report, Atlanta, GA: Author.

Centers for Disease Control and Prevention (CDC) (2001), *Taking action to combat increases in STDs and HIV risk among men who have sex with men*. Atlanta, GA: Author.

Cheuvront, J.P. (2002), High-risk sexual behavior in the treatment of HIV-negative patients. *J. Gay & Lesbian Psychotherapy*, 6(3):7-25.

Ciesielski C.A. (2003), Sexually transmitted diseases in men who have sex with men: An epidemiological review. *Current Infectious Disease Reports*, 5:145-152.

Drescher, J. (2002), Editorial: Barebacking: Psychotherapeutic and public health considerations. *J. Gay & Lesbian Psychotherapy*, 6(3):1-6.

Forstein, M. (2002), Commentary on Cheuvront's "High-risk sexual behavior in the treatment of HIV-negative patients." *J. Gay & Lesbian Psychotherapy*, 6(3):35-43.

Gendin, S. (1997), Riding bareback; skin-on-skin sex–Been there, done that, want more. *Poz*, June, pp. 64-65.

Goodroad, B.K., Kirksey, K.M. & Butensky, E. (2000), Bareback sex and gay men: An HIV prevention failure. *J. Association Nurses in AIDS Care*, 11(6):29-36.

Green, J. (1996), Flirting with suicide. *The New York Times Magazine*, September 15, pp. 39-45, 54-55, 85-85.

Halkitis, P.N. (2001), An exploration of perceptions of masculinity among gay men living with HIV. *J. Men's Studies*, 9(3):413-429.

Halkitis, P.N. & Parsons, J.T. (1998), Drawing conclusions on barebacking. *The New York Blade*. September 11, 2(37), p. 19.

Halkitis, P.N. & Parsons, J.T. (2003), Intentional unsafe sex (barebacking) among men who meet sexual partners on the Internet. *AIDS Care*, 15(3):367-378.

Halkitis, P.N., Parsons, J.T. & Wilton, L. (2003), Barebacking, among gay and bisexual men in New York City. *Archives Sexual Behavior*, 32(4):351-358.

Halkitis, P.N., Wilton, L., Wolitski, R.J., Parsons, J.T., Hoff, C. & Bimbi, D. (2005), Barebacking identity among HIV-positive gay and bisexual men: Demographic, psychological, and behavioral correlates. *AIDS(*suppl*)*: 527-538.

Jost S., Bernard M.C., Kaiser L., Yerly S., Hirschel B., Samri A., Autran B., Goh L.E. & Perrin L. (2002), A patient with HIV-1 superinfection. *New England J. Medicine*, 347:731-736.

Koblin, B.A., Torian, L.V., Gulin, V., Ren, L., MacKellar, D.A. & Valleroy, L.A. (2000), High prevalence of HIV infection among young men who have sex with men in New York City. *AIDS*, 14:1793-1800.

Mansergh, G., Marks, G., Colfax, G., Guzman, R., Rader, M. & Buchbinder, S. (2002), Barebacking in a diverse sample of men who have sex with men. *AIDS*. 16:653-659.

Orange, D. (2002), High-risk behavior or high-risk systems? Discussion of Chuevront's "High-risk sexual behavior in the treatment of HIV-negative patient." *J. Gay & Lesbian Psychotherapy*, 6(3):45-50

Rotello, G. (1997), *Sexual Ecology: AIDS and the Destiny of Men*. New York: Dutton.

Shilts, R. (1987), *And The Band Played On*. New York: St. Martin's Press.

Valdiserri, R.O. (2003). *Preventing New HIV Infections in the US: What Can We Hope to Achieve?* Paper presented at the 10th Conference on Retroviruses and Opportunistic Infections, Boston, US, February.

Valleroy, L., MacKellar, D.A., Karon, J.M., Rosen, D.H., MacFarland, W., Shehan, D.A., Stoyanoff, S.R., LaLota, M., Celentano, D.D., Koblin, B.A., Thiede, H., Katz, M.H., Torian, L.V. & Janssen, R.S. (2000), HIV prevalence and associated risks in young men who have sex with men. *JAMA*, 282(2):198-204.

Vernazza, P.L., Bernasconi, E. & Hirschel, B. (2000), HIV superinfection: Myth or reality. *Schweiz. Med. Wochenschr.*, 130(31-32):1101-1104.

Whitmore, S.K., Zaidi, I.F., Dean, H.D., Hu, S. & Gerstle, J.E. (2004), *Concurrent Diagnoses of HIV Infection among Women Infected Through Heterosexual Contact in 30 Areas, 1999-2001, United States*. Paper presented at the XV International Aids Conference, Bangkok, Thailand, July.

Wiley D.J., Visscher B.R., Grosser, S., Hoover, D.R., Day, R., Gange, S., et al. (2000), Evidence that anoreceptive intercourse with ejaculate exposure is associated with rapid CD4 loss. *AIDS*, 14:707-715.

Wolitski, R.J., Valdiserri, R.O., Denning, P.H. & Levine, W.C. (2001), Are we headed for a resurgence in the HIV epidemic among men who have sex with men? *American J. Public Health*, 91:883-888.

The Emergence of Barebacking Among Gay and Bisexual Men in the United States: A Public Health Perspective

Richard J. Wolitski, PhD

SUMMARY. Barebacking (intentional unprotected anal sex) represents a significant threat to the health of gay, bisexual, and other men who have sex with men (MSM), which is not well defined and understood. Despite a relative lack of research on this issue, most MSM have heard of barebacking, and a substantial minority has had bareback sex. Individual reasons and six community-level influences that may have contributed to the emergence of barebacking are reviewed: (1) improvements in HIV treatment, (2) more complex sexual decision-making, (3) the Internet, (4) substance use, (5) safer sex fatigue, and (6) changes in HIV prevention programs. The implications of barebacking for

Richard J. Wolitski is Acting Chief, Prevention Research Branch, Division of HIV/AIDS Prevention, National Center for HIV, STD, and TB Prevention, Centers for Disease Control and Prevention.

Address correspondence to: Richard J. Wolitski, PRB, DHAP, NCHSTP, CDC, 1600 Clifton Road (MS E-37), Atlanta, GA 30333 (E-mail: RWolitski@cdc.gov).

The author would like to thank Ron Stall, Ron Valdiserri, Linda Valleroy, and the editors of the special issue for their helpful feedback and Jill Wasserman for her assistance with identifying and obtaining the reference materials for this paper.

[Haworth co-indexing entry note]: "The Emergence of Barebacking Among Gay and Bisexual Men in the United States: A Public Health Perspective." Wolitski, Richard J. Co-published simultaneously in *Journal of Gay & Lesbian Psychotherapy* (The Haworth Medical Press, an imprint of The Haworth Press, Inc.) Vol. 9, No. 3/4, 2005, pp. 9-34; and: *Barebacking: Psychosocial and Public Health Approaches* (ed: Perry N. Halkitis, Leo Wilton, and Jack Drescher) The Haworth Medical Press, an imprint of The Haworth Press, Inc., 2005, pp. 9-34. Single or multiple copies of this article are available for a fee from The Haworth Document Delivery Service [1-800-HAWORTH, 9:00 a.m. - 5:00 p.m. (EST). E-mail address: docdelivery@haworthpress.com].

Available online at http://www.haworthpress.com/web/JGLP
doi:10.1300/J236v09n03_02

HIV prevention are discussed, and suggestions for future research are offered. *[Article copies available for a fee from The Haworth Document Delivery Service: 1-800-HAWORTH. E-mail address: <docdelivery@haworthpress.com> Website: <http://www.HaworthPress.com>]*

KEYWORDS. Barebacking, bisexual, gay, HIV/AIDS prevention, homosexuality, human immunodeficiency virus, MSM, psychosexual behavior, safer sex, sexual risk taking, STI

Accurately identifying a new behavioral or epidemiological trend is often difficult. Small increases in risk behavior or disease incidence can signify the beginning of what may become a dramatic shift that affects an entire population. Alternatively, these increases may merely represent normal variation, measurement error, or change in a small segment of a community that will ultimately fail to affect a large number of persons.

A number of years ago, three colleagues and I wrote an article that assessed whether we were facing a resurgence of the HIV epidemic among gay and bisexual men (Wolitski et al., 2001). We reviewed evidence indicating that an increase in HIV infections might be on the horizon–sexually transmitted infections (STIs) among gay, bisexual and other men who have sex with men (MSM) had risen in a number of cities, beliefs about HIV treatment had caused some men to be more willing to engage in unprotected sex, and data from San Francisco showed increases in unprotected anal intercourse. At that time, rates of HIV infection appeared to be relatively stable, and there was no compelling evidence that an increase in HIV transmission had accompanied these changes in self-reported sexual practices and STI rates.

Since that time, additional outbreaks of STIs have been reported (Ciesielski, 2003), and HIV diagnoses have begun to increase among MSM for the first time in nearly two decades. In the 25 states that have reported HIV cases for 10 or more years, new HIV diagnoses among MSM increased nearly 18% between 1999 and 2002 (Jaffe, 2003). Small increases in HIV incidence have also been observed among MSM seeking anonymous HIV testing in San Francisco. From 1996 to 1999, annual HIV incidence among MSM increased from 2.1% to 4.2% in testing sites, and remained stable at 5.3% in STI clinics (Katz et al., 2002).

These data provide compelling evidence that a growing number of MSM are not consistently maintaining safer sex practices. What the data do not do, however, is provide the insights that are necessary to develop effective interventions that protect the health of gay, bisexual, and other MSM. A large number of studies have examined characteristics that affect risk behavior among MSM, and reviews of this literature (Hospers and Kok, 1995; Stall et al., 2000) provide a useful starting point for understanding why some men engage in behaviors that put them at risk for HIV and STIs. Undoubtedly, many of the same individual, social, and structural factors that have influenced risk behavior since the beginning of the HIV epidemic (i.e., substance use, social and behavioral norms, assumptions about partners' HIV serostatus, condom availability, etc.) remain critically important today. This body of research is important because it promotes an understanding of why some men engage in unprotected sex and others do not. What the research does not do, however, is clarify why, at this particular point in time, some MSM are now more willing to engage in risky sexual practices than they were in the past.

The articles in this issue of the *Journal of Gay & Lesbian Psychotherapy* provide important insights into a new phenomenon–barebacking–that has emerged among gay and bisexual men in the past 6-8 years. In the present context of the HIV epidemic, barebacking represents much more than a return of unprotected sexual practices that were the norm prior to the diagnosis of the first AIDS cases. The emergence of barebacking may be viewed as both a symptom and a cause of broader changes in the ways that MSM think about HIV, their risk of becoming infected or infecting someone else, and the physical, mental, and social consequences of being HIV-positive. Barebacking may be a *symptom* that is the result of the availability of highly active antiretroviral therapy (HAART), changes in how prevention programs are conducted, and other changes in the gay community. It may also be a *cause* of increased risk by providing a social identity for men who prefer unprotected sex, creating role models that celebrate the benefits of unprotected sex, changing social norms about protected and unprotected sexual practices, and establishing social and sexual networks of men who prefer unprotected sex. Before delving into these issues further, it is necessary to more clearly define barebacking and the ways in which it is different from other types of unprotected sex.

BAREBACKING DEFINED

The meaning of the word "barebacking" has evolved over time. At its core, barebacking describes unprotected anal intercourse among MSM (Yep, Lovaas and Pagonis, 2002). The term is not applied to unprotected oral sex, which carries a much lower risk of HIV transmission (Rothenberg et al., 1998; Wolitski and Branson, 2002). In most instances, the term is reserved for acts in which unprotected or "raw" sex was desired and intentional. This element of conscious intentionality is a critical element of barebacking that differentiates it from episodic lapses or "slips" among persons who otherwise strive to maintain safer sex practices. As such, the emergence of barebacking does not merely indicate that a greater number of men are having a harder time maintaining safer sex practices. Rather, it reflects the fact that a growing number of MSM have consciously rejected condom-protected sex in some, or all, circumstances.

The willingness to accept or seek out risk in a sexual encounter is another key element of barebacking. Men who have bareback sex face varied risks depending on whether they are HIV-positive or uninfected. Uninfected men who bareback risk HIV infection and exposure to other STIs. HIV-positive barebackers risk exposure to STIs that may adversely affect their health (O'Brien et al., 1999; Wiley et al., 2000), the possibility of reinfection with other strains of HIV (Blackard, Cohen and Mayer, 2002; Halkitis et al., 2004), and the potential social, legal, and psychological consequences associated with exposing partners to HIV. Infection with an STI also increases the ability of HIV-infected individuals to transmit HIV and makes uninfected persons more susceptible to infection (Fleming and Wasserheit, 1999).

For some men, the risks associated with barebacking may be an integral part of what makes the behavior appealing to them (Crossley, 2002; Davis, 2002). The most extreme examples of this perspective come from a small number of accounts that describe uninfected men who actively search for multiple HIV-positive partners ("bug chasers") in the hope of becoming infected (Gauthier and Forsyth, 1999). Other men seek to manage the risks associated with barebacking by only having unprotected sex with partners whose HIV status is perceived to be the same as their own, limiting the number of bareback partners, withdrawing prior to ejaculation, or adopting other behaviors that they believe will reduce the risk of acquiring or transmitting an unwanted infection (Scarce, 1999; Schwartz and Bailey, 2005; Suarez and Miller, 2001; Van de Ven et al., 2002). These men may have considered the risks associated with unprotected anal intercourse and decided that the risks involved are unlikely, not very serious, or for some HIV-positive MSM, inconsequential compared to the effects of already having HIV (Gold, Skinner and Ross, 1994; Schwartz and Bailey, 2005; Suarez and Miller, 2001).

Although some men who bareback may adopt strategies to manage the risk associated with this behavior, it is important to differentiate barebacking from risk management strategies that specifically seek to balance the long-term avoidance of HIV infection against the pleasures of unprotected sex. For HIV-negative persons, having sex within a mutually monogamous relationship with an uninfected partner is one such strategy. In Australia, the practice of "negotiated safety" has been widely promoted as a safer sex strategy for nearly a decade (Kippax, 2002). There are five conditions that must be met in a negotiated safety relationship:

1. The sexual partners are in an on-going primary relationship;
2. The sexual partners are HIV-antibody negative and aware of each other's negative antibody status;
3. The sexual partners have reached a clear and unambiguous agreement about the types of sexual behaviors that will be practiced within and outside of their relationship;
4. The agreement is that sex outside of the relationship is safe with regard to HIV transmission; and
5. The agreement is kept by all partners.

Unprotected anal sex that occurs between two uninfected men cannot lead to HIV transmission and can be an efficacious HIV risk reduction strategy if mutual monogamy or negotiated safety can be established and maintained. Unprotected anal sex that occurs outside of these relationships does not provide the same protection, and significantly increases gay and bisexual men's risk of HIV and other STIs.

Mansergh and colleagues (2002) have proposed a definition of barebacking that addresses many of these issues and differentiates barebacking from other forms of unprotected anal sex. They defined barebacking as: "intentional anal sex without a condom with men who are not a primary partner" (p. 654). This definition addresses the intentionality of the behavior, limits the practice to unprotected anal intercourse, and excludes unprotected sex that may occur within a mutually monogamous relationship or negotiated safety relationship. Although this may be the most parsimonious and easily understood definition that can be achieved, it excludes some types of intentional unprotected anal intercourse that should be accommodated by a public health definition of barebacking: unprotected anal sex between serodiscordant primary partners, unprotected anal sex between seroconcordant primary partners who have unprotected sex outside of their relationship, and unprotected sex between HIV-positive primary seroconcordant partners. All of these relationships present a risk that one partner may transmit HIV or another STI to the other.

An alternative, although somewhat cumbersome, definition that encompasses these complexities is: "intentional anal sex without a condom except when practiced by HIV-negative primary partners who maintain a mutually monogamous or negotiated safety relationship with each other." Using this definition, all intentional unprotected anal intercourse between non-primary partners (regardless of HIV status) and unprotected anal intercourse between serodiscordant primary partners and seroconcordant HIV-positive primary partners would fit within the definition of barebacking. The importance of this definition for public health is that it avoids confusing barebacking with unprotected anal intercourse between two HIV-negative partners in a protective relationship (i.e., mutual monogamy, negotiated safety), thus clearly differentiating behaviors that promote risk from those that reduce risk.

PREVALENCE OF BAREBACKING

Barebacking has become a familiar term among urban gay men, and a significant minority of MSM now report engaging in bareback sex. In San Francisco, 70% of 554 men interviewed from mid-2000 to early-2001 indicated that they had heard of barebacking (Mansergh et al., 2002), and 86% of 518 men in a New York City study were familiar with the term (Halkitis, Parsons and Wilton, 2003a). Not surprisingly, the way that researchers define barebacking can dramatically affect the number of men who report engaging in the behavior. In the New York City study, barebacking was not defined and men who were aware of the term used their own definition for it. Of the 448 men in this study who were familiar with barebacking, nearly half (46%) reported that they had bareback sex in the past three months. In the San Francisco study, fewer men reported engaging in barebacking when the behavior was defined as intentional unprotected anal intercourse with a non-primary partner. Using this definition, 14% of the 390 men who were aware of barebacking reported engaging in the behavior in the past two years.

Despite differences in how barebacking was defined, both studies found that HIV-positive MSM were more likely to have bareback sex than were HIV-negative MSM. Mansergh and colleagues reported that

HIV-positive and negative men in San Francisco were equally likely to have heard of barebacking (72% of 138 men versus 70% of 239 men, respectively), but more HIV-positive men (22%) reported engaging in this behavior than did HIV-seronegative men (10%). Halkitis, Parsons and Wilton also found that HIV-positive MSM in New York were more likely than HIV-negative men to engage in barebacking (61% of 87 men versus 42% of 361 men), and that HIV-positive men reported a larger number of bareback sex partners than did HIV-negative men. For many men, HIV serostatus also appears to influence with whom they have bareback sex. HIV-positive men who bareback are more likely to report that they had unprotected anal intercourse with a partner who was also HIV-positive than they are to report having had unprotected anal intercourse with partners who are HIV-negative or whose serostatus they do not know (Mansergh et al., 2002). Similarly, HIV-negative men are more likely to report having unprotected anal intercourse with a partner who was HIV-negative or of unknown serostatus than a partner who was known to be HIV-positive (Mansergh et al., 2002). This pattern of findings suggests at least some attempt on the part of these MSM to minimize HIV transmission during bareback sex.

However, many barebackers do not limit unprotected anal sex to only those partners whose HIV status is the same as their own. One study found that the majority of HIV-positive MSM in New York City and San Francisco who bareback did not limit these encounters to other HIV-positive men (Halkitis et al., 2005). Among the 316 HIV-positive MSM in this study who identified themselves as barebackers, more than half (57%) reported that they had bareback sex with partners who were HIV-negative or whose serostatus they did not know. Another study asked men in San Francisco who bareback about their last bareback sex encounter (Mansergh et al., 2002). Fourteen percent of 29 HIV-positive barebackers had unprotected insertive anal intercourse (the sexual behavior most likely to transmit HIV to an uninfected partner) with an HIV-negative partner, and 24% said they engaged in this behavior with a partner whose HIV status they did not know. When the 23 HIV-negative barebackers were asked the same question, 17% reported that they had unprotected receptive anal intercourse (the sexual behavior that places an uninfected person at greatest risk of becoming infected) with a partner they knew was HIV-positive, and 43% had done so with a partner whose HIV status they did not know. Barebacking with a known serodiscordant partner represents a willingness to risk infection. Barebacking with a partner of unknown status may involve misperception of the risks involved that are affected by assumptions about partner serostatus.

When direct communication about serostatus does not occur, some men make assumptions about the HIV status of their partners that often leads them to believe that their partner's serostatus is the same as their own (Gold and Skinner, 1996; Gold, Skinner and Hinchy, 1999; Suarez and Miller, 2001). That is, HIV-negative men look for cues that are consistent with a desire to believe that their partner is uninfected. HIV-positive men often use similar cues to infer that their partner is HIV-positive. These assumptions provide a rationale for unsafe behaviors that may serve to justify desired sex acts during a sexual encounter or reduce anxiety or guilt following unsafe sexual encounters.

THE EMERGENCE OF BAREBACKING

In order to facilitate the adoption of healthier behaviors among MSM who bareback, it is important to understand why some individuals choose to engage in this behavior and others do not. This level of understanding is critical to the success of individual counseling to reduce the risk of clients whose behavior places themselves or others at risk for HIV infection. It is also important to consider how broader community-level changes may have shaped individuals' motivations and led to shifts in the perceptions and behavior of large numbers of MSM.

Individual Reasons for Barebacking

A rapidly growing number of studies has examined correlates of unprotected sex among persons living with HIV (for review see Crepaz and Marks, 2002). Very few studies have specifically addressed motivations for engaging in bareback sex. The existing literature largely consists of case reports, small qualitative studies, and syntheses of information published from scientific journals, the popular press, and the Internet (i.e., Cheuvront, 2002; Crossley, 2002; Davis, 2002; Gauthier and Forsyth, 1999; Goodroad, Kirksey and Butensky, 2000; Halkitis, Parsons and Wilton, 2003a; Yep, Lovaas and Pagonis, 2002). One of the larger studies asked 53 barebackers in San Francisco to give up to three reasons for having bareback sex (Mansergh et al., 2002). The reason most frequently endorsed was to experience greater physical stimulation (80% of HIV-positive MSM and 65% of HIV-negative men). The second most frequently mentioned reason was to feel emotionally closer or a sense of connection with a sex partner (40% of HIV-positive MSM and 39% of HIV-negative men). A desire to rebel against established norms (i.e., to do something taboo or "racy") was the third most frequently endorsed reason for barebacking among HIV-positive (10%) and HIV-negative men (17%). Dislike of condoms was also endorsed by 17% of HIV-negative men, but was cited by only 7% of HIV-positive men. It is important to note that this early study may not have adequately captured men's reasons for engaging in bareback sex–43% of HIV-positive and 35% of HIV-negative men indicated another reason for barebacking that was not specified by the researchers.

Community-Level Reasons for Barebacking

Given that there are few data on individual-level reasons for barebacking, it is not surprising that even less is known about the effects of broader community-level influences that may have contributed to the emergence of barebacking. These social, structural, and technological influences exist outside of the individual and can influence the attitudes and behavior of large numbers of individuals (Sumartojo, 2000; Wolitski et al., 2004). Identifying community-level influences may not explain why a given individual has bareback sex, but considering these factors may provide insight into the reasons that substantial numbers of men have decided to actively reject condom use at this particular point in time. Potential community-level influences have been identified by Halkitis, Parsons and Wilton (2003a) who assessed reasons for the emergence of barebacking among 204 MSM from New York City who reported engaging in this behavior. More than two-thirds of participants endorsed items addressing a link between barebacking and substance use and meeting sex partners on the internet. Slightly fewer than half of these men also indicated that they believed barebacking had emerged because of "boring" safer sex campaigns (49%), improvements in HIV treatment (48%), and a sense of fatigue from dealing with AIDS-related issues for so long (46%). In addition, some researchers have suggested that increases in unprotected anal sex among MSM may reflect complex sexual decision making based on scientific evidence rather than a greater willingness to risk HIV infection (i.e., Kippax and Race, 2003; Van de Ven et al., 2002). The evidence supporting these reasons is reviewed below.

Improvements in HIV Treatment. In the last decade there have been significant advances in HIV treatment that have changed the course of the epidemic and how it is perceived. The availability of HAART and treatments to prevent opportunistic infections have significantly improved the quantity and quality of life for many persons with HIV. The development of viral load tests that measure levels of HIV in the blood has significantly improved the ability of physicians to monitor disease progression and to make better informed decisions about initiating or changing HIV treatments. Considered together, these advances have greatly benefited HIV-positive persons by dramatically slowing the progression of HIV disease and reducing HIV-related deaths (Centers for Disease Control and Prevention [CDC], 2001a). As a result of these advances, the number of persons living with HIV has grown in recent years. In 2000, an estimated 850,000-950,000 persons were living with HIV in the United States (US) (Fleming et al., 2002).

The growing number of sexually active persons living with HIV increases the probability that uninfected MSM will have partners who are HIV-positive, and has led public health agencies to place a greater emphasis on encouraging the adoption and maintenance of safer sex practices among people living with HIV (CDC, 2003; Janssen et al., 2001). Most persons living with HIV reduce sexual practices that can transmit HIV after they are diagnosed with the virus (Weinhardt et al., 1999; Wolitski et al., 1997). About one-third, however, engage in sexual practices that present at least some risk of HIV transmission (Marks, Burris and Peterman, 1999). For some HIV-positive MSM, using condoms is an uncomfortable reminder of their HIV status, serves to separate them physically and emotionally from their partners, and contributes to feelings of shame and guilt about having HIV (Remien, Carballo-Dieguez and Wagner, 1995). Having sex without condoms can represent an effort to avoid these feelings and may be perceived by some MSM as a "consolation prize" or "membership privilege" that is afforded those who no longer have to worry about contracting HIV (Yep, Lovaas and Pagonis, 2002).

Advances in HIV treatment may also have had more widespread effects on the sexual behavior of MSM by decreasing the perceived severity and consequences of HIV transmission. Positive beliefs about the effects of HAART may contribute to (or serve as a justification for) increased sexual risk taking among a small percentage of MSM (Dilley, Woods and McFarland, 1997; Kalichman et al., 1998; Kelly et al., 1998; Vanable et al., 2000). For example, one study found that 26% of gay men reported that because of new treatments they were much less concerned about becoming HIV-positive, and 15% indicated that they had already taken a chance of getting infected (Dilley, Woods and McFarland, 1997). It is important to note that the effects of beliefs about HAART may vary in different communities (International Collaboration on HIV Optimism, 2003), and that important questions about the causal influence of treatment beliefs on risk behavior have not yet been resolved (Elford, Bolding and Sherr, 2001b).

Knowledge of one's own (or a sex partner's) viral load may also influence beliefs about the risk of HIV transmission and risk behavior (Kalichman et al., 2001; Kelly et al., 1998). These beliefs are not entirely irrational–one study has found that low viral load may decrease heterosexual HIV transmission (Quinn et al., 2000), suggesting that HIV treatment may reduce the transmissibility of HIV at a population level. Caution is warranted, however, because some men with an undetectable plasma viral load may still have detectable virus in their semen, and the amount of HIV in semen can vary over time as a result of poor adherence, treatment interruption, treatment failure, and other factors (Barroso et al., 2000, 2003; Tubiana et al., 2002). Furthermore, HAART-related decreases in the transmissibility of HIV can be offset by increases in unprotected sex (Blower et al., 2000; Katz et al., 2002). Thus, the HIV epidemic can expand even if HIV treatments lead to community-level reductions in viral load and decrease the transmissibility of HIV. These data reinforce the need to encourage HIV-positive persons and their partners to maintain safer sex practices regardless of whether they are receiving HIV treatment or their viral load is undetectable.

Evidence-Based Sexual Decision Making. Kippax and Race (2003) have suggested that increases in unprotected sex among MSM may reflect a greater reliance on complex sexual decision making that is informed by accumulating scientific evidence about the dynamics of HIV transmission. This use of scientific data about HIV transmission goes beyond awareness of research findings on the effects of HIV treatment and viral load, and includes information about the relative risk of specific sexual practices and partner serostatus. Kippax and Race argue that MSM have not become less concerned about HIV, but that they are making increasingly complex and rational decisions about the sexual practices in which they are willing to engage. A growing body of evidence supports the idea that MSM are adopting harm reduction strategies that are based on the HIV status of their partner and the relative risk of specific sexual practices (for review see Wolitski and Branson, 2002). As previously described, barebackers are more likely to report having had unprotected sex with partners whose HIV status was the same as their own than with partners who were serodiscordant, which limits the risk of HIV transmission to uninfected partners (Halkitis, Parsons and Wilton, 2003a; Mansergh et al., 2002). Van de Ven and colleagues (2002) provide additional evidence that information about HIV serostatus and the relative risks of insertive versus receptive anal intercourse is being used by some MSM to manage HIV risk. They have labeled this pattern of risk management behavior "strategic positioning." Their research with MSM in Australia indicates that some HIV-positive MSM are more likely to adopt the receptive role during unprotected anal intercourse with HIV-negative partners than they are with HIV-positive partners. On the other hand, HIV-negative men are more likely to adopt the insertive role with partners they know are HIV positive than with seroconcordant partners. These same patterns are not observed, however, for condom-protected sex. This further strengthens the argument that some MSM are making decisions that are influenced by partner serostatus and the risk of HIV transmission when deciding to forgo condoms. Qualitative research with HIV-positive men also provides evidence for the use of strategic positioning based on partner serostatus and the adoption of other risk management strategies (such as withdrawing prior to ejaculation) that are based on an understanding of empirical data and reasoned assumptions about the dynamics of HIV transmission (Schwartz and Bailey, 2005).

The Internet. Technological advances outside of medicine have also affected the sexual practices of MSM and may have contributed to the emergence of barebacking. In the past decade, the Internet has created new opportunities for MSM to meet sex partners. The Internet is available 24 hours a day, 7 days a week, and makes it possible for users to anonymously identify their sexual interests and to find partners with similar sexual interests without having to leave the house (Bull and McFarlane, 2000). Sexually explicit websites, including those that are designed primarily for MSM who are looking for sex, have proliferated on the Internet. Websites that are dedicated to helping people find romantic or sexual partners allow users to post their photograph and personal profiles that describe themselves and the attributes they are seeking in a sex partner. Thousands of profiles can be quickly searched to identify partners by location, physical and demographic characteristics, and preferred sexual practices. These sites allow men to identify their preference for unprotected sex either by selecting from a pull-down menu of pre-selected options (i.e., safer sex only, needs further discussion) or by describing their preference for protected or unprotected sex in their personal profiles by including keywords such as "safe only," "bareback," "bb," or "raw."

A small number of sites have also been created specifically for men who are looking for bareback sex partners (i.e., barebacksex.com, barebackcity.com). These sites allow men to disclose their HIV status if they choose and to identify potential partners based on their serostatus. The ability to search for sex partners on the Internet makes it possible for men who want to have bareback sex to find like-minded partners without risking in-person rejection or critical interpersonal feedback for attempting to violate safer sex recommendations. It creates new sexual and social networks by establishing connections between men who might not otherwise know that they share a desire to have unprotected sex. The Internet has also made this private behavior much more public, creating awareness among other gay men that some of their peers have rejected safer sex, which is likely to contribute to the erosion of safer sex norms by providing informal role models who embrace the pleasures and accept the risks of unprotected sex.

Many MSM now use the Internet to meet sex partners. Thirty-four percent of 609 men in a community-based sample in Atlanta had met one or more sex partners via the Internet (Benotsch, Kalichman and Cage, 2002). Men who use the Internet to meet sex partners may be at elevated risk for acquiring or transmitting HIV and other STIs. Compared to MSM who do not meet sex partners on the Internet, MSM who meet sex partners online report having more sex partners, and are more likely to use methamphetamines, have unprotected anal sex, have sex with an HIV-positive partner, and to have had an STI in the prior year (Benotsch, Kalichman and Cage, 2002; Elford, Bolding and Sherr, 2001a; Kim et al., 2001). Use of online chat rooms to meet sex partners has also been linked to at least one syphilis outbreak (Klausner et al., 2000).

Substance Use. Rates of substance use are elevated among MSM compared to other community-based samples of men (Stall et al., 2001), and increases in MSM's use of some recreational drugs have coincided with increases in unprotected sex and the advent of barebacking (Halkitis et al., 2005). It is not known whether a common influence has led to a relaxation of social prohibitions against drug use and risky sex or if changes in substance use have contributed to increases in unprotected sex. Of particular concern is the increase in methamphetamine use, which has reached epidemic proportions in the western and midwestern US and has spread to other areas of the country (National Institute on Drug Abuse, 1998; Rawson, Anglin and Ling, 2002).

Methamphetamine (commonly referred to as "crystal" or "Tina") is often used to lower sexual inhibitions, enhance sexual encounters, and extend their duration (Frosch et al., 1996; Halkitis, Parsons and Wilton, 2003b). Methamphetamine is considered a "club" or "party" drug along with ecstasy, ketamine, and GHB. Club drugs are commonly used in dance venues (such as bars and circuit parties) and to enhance sexual experiences. These drugs, along with alcohol and nitrate inhalants or "poppers," have been associated with risky sexual practices among MSM (Halkitis, Parsons and Stirratt, 2001; Purcell et al., 2001; Romanelli, Smith and Pomeroy, 2003; Stall and Purcell, 2000). The use of these drugs is especially prevalent at rave-like circuit parties, which increased in popularity and number in the 1990s (Colfax et al., 2001; Mansergh et al., 2001). Attendance at circuit parties, particularly those that required out of town travel, has been associated with increased levels of unprotected sex among HIV-positive and HIV-negative MSM (Coflax et al., 2001; Mansergh et al., 2001).

Safer Sex Fatigue and HIV Prevention Programs. Long-term effort to maintain safer sex practices, repeated exposure to prevention messages, and the loss of many loved ones to AIDS may contribute to a decreased ability or unwillingness on the part of some MSM to attend to HIV-related issues. This phenomenon is known as "safer sex fatigue" or "AIDS burnout." A four-city study indicates that safer sex fatigue is an independent predictor of risky sexual practices among HIV-positive MSM. In this study of 547 men, those who scored higher on a measure of safer sex fatigue were more likely to report unprotected anal intercourse (Ostrow et al., 2002).

The challenges of maintaining MSM's interest in prevention efforts may be exacerbated by a failure of some HIV prevention programs to update risk reduction messages, develop new approaches to prevention, and meet the evolving needs of a diverse community. Criticisms of HIV prevention programs for MSM have included a failure to speak to the needs of communities at greatest risk and providing outdated or overly simplistic prevention messages for MSM that fail to take partner serostatus and risk management strategies into account (Gold, 1995; Kippax and Race, 2003; Odets, 1994; Rotello, 1997; Wilton, 2001). It is possible that these issues may have reduced the salience of HIV in the minds of some MSM, alienated them, or contributed to the perception that these programs are not in touch with the current needs and concerns of MSM.

Although empirical data do not exist, it is possible that changes in the way that HIV prevention programs are conducted have also contributed to the emergence of barebacking. Although the messages that HIV prevention programs provide to MSM have remained relatively unchanged, the manner in which these programs are conducted has changed profoundly in the past decade. In the early years of the epidemic, HIV prevention programs were largely the result of grass-roots efforts that emerged from within the gay community (Kippax and Race, 2003; Reverson and Schiaffino, 2000; Shilts, 1987). Members of the gay community came together to advocate for resources to care for persons who were sick, fight the stigma associated with AIDS, and volunteer their time to educate themselves and their community about the disease and its prevention. At the time, many also came together to voice their anger about the government's response to the epidemic. There were few financial resources for AIDS care and prevention efforts, and many believed at the time that if the gay community did not mobilize to respond to the epidemic, no one else would. In that context, the adoption of safer sex strategies represented both a personal strategy for protecting one's own health and a political action against a society that seemed indifferent to the suffering of persons with AIDS and the spread of the epidemic within the gay community.

Funding for HIV-related research and services has dramatically increased and has spawned an industry that is supported by hundreds of millions of local, state, and federal dollars each year. Although many HIV-prevention programs still rely on volunteers, these programs are now largely staffed by paid personnel. As the impact of the HIV epidemic has broadened, prevention efforts have been expanded to meet the needs of other populations, and potential gaps in HIV prevention services for MSM have developed (Aral, 1999).

The staff and the client base of many of these HIV prevention programs have also changed to reflect the diverse populations they serve. These changes have "de-gayed" the HIV epidemic in the minds of some MSM and have changed the way in which some local agencies and the services they provide are perceived (Rotello, 1997). Some organizations that were once seen as a part of the gay community may no longer be viewed, or perceive themselves, in this way. These fundamental changes in how (and by whom) HIV prevention is conducted may have resulted in a perception among some MSM that HIV prevention does not represent their needs or represents an attempt by the government and other outsiders (labeled the "condomocracy" by one commentator) to control and dictate the sexual practices of gay and bisexual men (Savage, 1999). The reactance of some gay men against HIV prevention has fomented a backlash in which some men are rebelling against what they perceive to be an overly antiseptic and puritanical view of sex that chastises MSM for their sexual desires and seeks to deny them the right to sexual pleasure (Crossley, 2002). This sense of rebellion against prevention and safer sex norms is reflected in the self-perception of some barebackers, which Blechner (2002) described as ". . . proud and defiant, in what some see as courageous behavior against sexual repression and punitive attitudes, sometimes tinged with homophobia" (p. 29).

CONCLUSION

Unprotected sex among gay and bisexual men is not a new phenomenon. Condom-less sex was the norm before the first AIDS cases were reported in 1981. At that time, most sexually transmitted infections were treatable and had relatively few long-term consequences. That is not to say that sex between men was without risk. The highly stigmatized nature of homosexuality led many men to seek partners in public sex environments that facilitated quick and anonymous encounters, but left them vulnerable to arrest or physical attack. The stigma associated with homosexuality meant that disclosing one's sexual orientation was likely to disrupt valued interpersonal relationships or lead to other social sanctions. Thus, living with the fact that their sexual practices may jeopardize their psychological, social, financial, or physical well being is not a new experience for MSM. This context has important implications for HIV prevention efforts. Prevention programs that are perceived as coming from outside of the gay community run the risk of being perceived by at least some MSM as thinly veiled attacks on the lifestyles of gay and bisexual men. Given that MSM have become accustomed to filtering out messages that often discourage them from having any type of sexual relationships with other men, is it reasonable to assume that they will always be receptive to messages that discourage them from having a specific type of sex?

This social context necessitates the active involvement and support of community members in HIV prevention efforts. Active community involvement in HIV prevention efforts has waned since the early days of the epidemic, and some MSM may have become complacent about HIV as a result of improved treatments, AIDS burnout, and other influences. Community leaders and prevention agencies need to find new ways to mobilize gay men and reinvigorate HIV prevention efforts at the grassroots level.

There is a critical need to maintain the salience of HIV and the need to limit the further spread of HIV in the gay community. Reminders of the importance of protecting oneself and others from HIV should be a consistent and permanent part of venues frequented by MSM. That is not to suggest that prevention programs should plaster the community with graphic reminders of the debilitating effects of HIV to scare men into action or trap them into lengthy safer sex discussions in social venues. More subtle approaches are needed to remind men that safer sex is valued by the gay community because it has important benefits for individuals and the community as a whole. Such reminders can be as simple as having free condoms readily available in gay bars (as they were early in the epidemic), and may serve as important cues to action. HIV prevention information, counseling, and HIV testing should be readily available in venues that are frequented by MSM and that are amenable to these activities. Prevention messages should recognize the racial/ethnic and social diversity of the gay community and be framed in ways that are appealing and speak to the experiences of MSM of color and other segments of the MSM community. These messages should be updated on a regular basis to ensure that they address changing perceptions and practices and reflect the best available scientific information (Kippax and Race, 2003). HIV prevention messages, like other forms of persuasive communications, have a shelf life and are destined to become monotonous and stale, if they are not frequently changed and updated to reflect new scientific information or changes in community perceptions, norms, and values. HIV prevention needs to take a closer look at how advertising companies update their messages and repeatedly repackage the same product in new ways to maintain consumers' interest.

In order to avoid confusion about the risks associated with barebacking, prevention agencies should make gay and bisexual men aware of the potential misunderstandings that different uses of the term barebacking can bring about. Differentiating the risks associated with barebacking from those associated with carefully reasoned risk reduction strategies that include unprotected sex between uninfected primary partners is critical. Widespread awareness that some MSM have decided to have unprotected anal sex may weaken existing safer sex norms, and men who do not engage in barebacking may view this behavior as more acceptable because they know that others are doing it. In order to counter shifts in perceived norms regarding safer sex, it is important that prevention programs provide role models that communicate the commitment of other men to safer sex and reinforce the importance of stopping the further spread of HIV to protect one's own health and the health of the community.

There is a need to better understand the motivations of HIV-positive and HIV-negative men who bareback. The reports reviewed in this paper suggest important differences between men who bareback and those who do not, but much more remains to be learned about the psychological, contextual, and cultural determinants that lead some men to adopt this behavior and others to avoid it. A considerable weakness of the current research is that the majority of research participants have been White, gay-identified MSM. Too little is currently known about the importance and dynamics of barebacking and other forms of unprotected anal sex among MSM of color. This is a serious gap given the increased rates of HIV infection among Black and Latino MSM (CDC, 2001a, 2001b). It is important to recognize that all barebackers are not reckless risk takers (Suarez and Miller, 2001), and much remains to be learned about differences in risk taking among men who bareback (i.e., those who only bareback with partners who are perceived to have the same HIV status, HIV-negative men who are consciously trying to become infected, and HIV-positive men who bareback with uninfected partners).

Given the complexity of some MSM's sexual decision making, there is a need for research to clarify the effectiveness of strategic positioning and other risk management strategies so that prevention programs can provide accurate information about these strategies and their ability to reduce HIV transmission. For example, some men may believe that barebacking with a casual sex partner who says that he is HIV-negative is a reasonable risk reduction strategy. At this time, we do not have adequate data to evaluate the relative effectiveness of this strategy, but there is reason to suspect that it may not be effective in populations with a high incidence of HIV infection. Among young MSM, 77% of those who tested HIV-positive incorrectly believed that they were uninfected (MacKellar et al., 2002). Most of these men had previously tested negative for HIV infection and assumed that they were at low risk of having HIV. These data provide a clear warning that a partner's belief that he is uninfected may not afford meaningful protection against HIV transmission. Risk reduction strategies based on partner serostatus should be limited to partners in a primary relationship (i.e., mutual monogamy, negotiated safety) in which the HIV status of both partners is documented by repeat HIV testing.

It is particularly important for HIV prevention efforts to understand the mental health needs of persons who are consciously trying to contract or transmit HIV. Motivations to harm oneself or others may have roots in psychological trauma that was experienced years earlier and may be compounded by substance abuse. For example, a history of childhood sexual abuse has been associated with risk taking among HIV-negative and HIV-positive MSM (Bartholow et al., 1994; O'Leary et al., 2003). The experience of childhood sexual abuse may interact synergistically with other mental health issues to increase HIV risk. MSM who have experienced a greater number of mental health issues (i.e., childhood sexual abuse, partner violence, depression, substance use) are more likely to engage in high-risk sexual practices and to be HIV-positive than are those who have experienced fewer of these problems (Stall et al., 2003). Coping with an HIV diagnosis may present additional challenges to adopting and maintaining safer sex practices. For example, men who believe that their infection was the responsibility of someone else (or that another person purposefully infected them) may be more willing to engage in risky sexual practices than are men who perceive themselves as responsible for their infection (Bingman, Marks and Crepaz, 2001). A clearer understanding of how mental health issues affect risk taking, and how these issues can be addressed in psychotherapeutic settings and public health interventions, continues to be needed.

Most prevention programs are based on health behavior models that emphasize individuals' desire to avoid adverse outcomes that affect them personally. These models can fall short, however, when MSM decide that the risks of unprotected sex are acceptable or that these risks are no longer applicable to them because they are already infected with HIV. There is a need to expand these models to incorporate other-focused motivations. These motivations include concern about the effect of unsafe sexual practices on sex partners, friends and family, and the gay community in general as well as a desire to uphold personal or ethical values (Nimmons and Folkman, 1999). For HIV-positive persons, beliefs about their personal responsibility to protect partners from becoming infected are strongly associated with the avoidance of high-risk sexual practices and may be particularly important to address in prevention programs for this population (Wolitski et al., 2003). Care should be taken, however, when using appeals based on personal responsibility. Failure to acknowledge the physical, psychological, and social risks of unprotected sex to persons living with HIV could trigger reactance to the message and further stigmatize persons living with HIV by mistakenly communicating a lack of concern for their own health and well-being (Marks, Burris, and Peterman, 1999).

The ability of the Internet to affect HIV and STI risk is now well documented. What remains to be seen, however, is how Internet technology might be used to promote positive changes in social norms and personal attitudes toward safer sex. The Internet has the ability to provide prevention information, referrals to services, and interactive interventions to a large number of individuals, anonymously, at times when it is most convenient for them, and at a relatively low cost (Bull, McFarlane and King, 2001; Kalichman et al., 2002). In addition, the Internet provides an opportunity to target information to demographically or behaviorally defined subgroups of gay and bisexual men (by placing information on sites serving specific subgroups or designing new sites specifically for these individuals) or to tailor information to the specific characteristics, needs, and interests of individual users. The interactivity of the Internet makes it amenable to the development of risk assessments and learning activities that can help individuals better understand the risks of specific sexual practices and to more accurately assess their own risk (Benotsch, Kalichman and Cage, 2002). The Internet also provides "venues" (such as chat rooms for men seeking sex partners) for reaching men who are at increased risk of acquiring or transmitting HIV or other STIs. Given the substantial number of MSM who meet sex partners via the Internet, HIV prevention efforts need to devote additional energy to adapting existing intervention strategies and developing new approaches that can be effective in cyberspace.

Despite the considerable successes that have been achieved in HIV treatment and prevention, we cannot forget the significant threat that the virus continues to pose to the health and well being of gay and bisexual men. More than 20 years since the first cases of AIDS were reported in the U.S., HIV infection continues to be a major health threat for gay and bisexual men. MSM represent an estimated 60% of men in the US who developed AIDS in 2001 (CDC, 2001a), but only comprise 5% to 7% of men in the U.S. (Binson et al., 1995; Rogers and Turner, 1991). HAART has not allowed gay and bisexual men in the U.S. to put the devastation of AIDS behind them–6,588 MSM died from AIDS-related causes in 2001 (CDC, 2001a), and a new generation of MSM is threatened. In major US cities, as many as 1 in 8 young MSM between the ages of 23 and 29 may already be infected with HIV (CDC, 2001b). These prevalence rates, recent increases in new HIV diagnoses among MSM, and the emergence of barebacking underscore the pressing need to reevaluate and reinvigorate HIV prevention efforts for gay, bisexual, and other MSM. Unless we act decisively as individuals and as a community, we may be destined to repeat the hard-earned lessons that the epidemic has already taught us for many years to come.

REFERENCES

Aral, S. (1999), Elimination and reintroduction of a sexually transmitted disease: Lesson to be learned? *American J. Public Health*, 98:995-997.

Barroso, P.F., Schechter, M., Gupta, P., Melo, M.F., Vieira, M., Murta, F.C., Souza, Y. & Harrison, L.H. (2000), Effect of antiretroviral therapy on HIV shedding in semen. *Annals Internal Medicine*, 133:280-284.

Barroso, P.F., Schechter, M., Gupta, P., Bresan, C., Bomfim, A. & Harrison, L.H. (2003), Adherence to antiretroviral therapy and persistence of HIV RNA in semen. *J. Acquired Immune Deficiency Syndromes*, 32:435-440.

Bartholow, B.N., Doll, L.S., Joy, D., Douglas, J.M., Bolan, G., Harrision, J.S., Moss, P.M. & McKirnan, D. (1994), Emotional, behavioral, and HIV risks associated with sexual abuse among adult homosexual and bisexual men. *Child Abuse & Neglect*, 18:747-761.

Benotsch, E.G., Kalichman, S. & Cage, M. (2002), Men who have met sex partners via the Internet: Prevalence, predictors, and implications for HIV prevention. *Archives Sexual Behavior*, 31:77-183.

Bingman, C.R., Marks, G. & Crepaz, N. (2001), Attribution about one's HIV infection and unsafe sex in seropositive men who have sex with men. *AIDS & Behavior*, 5:283-289.

Binson, D., Michaels, S., Stall, R., Coates, T.J., Gagnon, J.H. & Catania, J.A. (1995), Prevalence and social distribution of men who have sex with men: United States and its urban centers. *J. Sex Research*, 32:245-254.

Blackard, J.T., Cohen, D.E. & Mayer, K.H. (2002), Human immunodeficiency virus superinfection and recombination: Current state of knowledge and potential clinical consequences. *Clinical Infectious Diseases*, 34:1108-1114.

Blechner, M.J. (2002), Intimacy, pleasure, risk, and safety: Discussion of Cheuvront's "High-risk sexual behavior in the treatment of HIV-negative patients." *J. Gay & Lesbian Psychotherapy*, 6:27-33.

Blower, S.M., Gershengorn, H.B. & Grant, R.M. (2000), A tale of two futures: HIV and antiretroviral therapy in San Francisco. *Science*, 287:650-654.

Bull, S.S. & McFarlane, M. (2000), Soliciting sex on the internet: What are the risks for sexually transmitted diseases and HIV? *Sexually Transmitted Diseases*, 27:545-550.

Bull, S.S., McFarlane, M., & King, D. (2001), Barriers to STD/HIV prevention on the Internet. *Health Education Research*, 16:661-670.

Centers for Disease Control and Prevention (2001a), *HIV/AIDS Surveillance Report*, 13:1-44.

Centers for Disease Control and Prevention (2001b). HIV incidence among young men who have sex with men–Seven U.S. cities, 1994-2000. *Morbidity & Mortality Weekly Report*, 50:440-444.

Centers for Disease Control and Prevention (2003), Advancing HIV prevention: New strategies for a changing epidemic–United States, 2003. *Morbidity & Mortality Weekly Report*, 52:329-332.

Cheuvront, J.P. (2002), High-risk sexual behavior in the treatment of HIV-negative patients. *J. Gay & Lesbian Psychotherapy*, 6:7-25.

Ciesielski, C.A. (2003), Sexually transmitted disease in men who have sex with men: An epidemiological review. *Current Infectious Disease Reports*, 5:145-152.

Colfax, G.N., Mansergh, G., Guzman, R., Vittinghoff, E., Marks, G., Rader, M. & Buchbinder, S. (2001), Drug use and sexual risk behavior among gay and bisexual men who attend circuit parties: A venue-based comparison. *J. Acquired Immune Deficiency Syndromes*, 28:373-379.

Crepaz, N. & Marks, G. (2002), Towards an understanding of sexual risk behavior in people living with HIV: A review of social, psychological, and medical findings. *AIDS*, 16:135-149.

Crossley, M.L. (2002), The perils of health promotion and the 'barebacking' backlash. *Health*, 6:47-68.

Davis, M. (2002), HIV prevention rationalities and serostatus in the risk narratives of gay men. *Sexualities*, 5:281-299.

Dilley, J.W., Woods, W.J. & McFarland, W. (1997), Are advances in treatment changing views about high-risk sex? *New England Journal Medicine*, 337:501-502.

Elford, J., Bolding, G. & Sherr, L. (2001a), Seeking sex on the Internet and sexual risk behavior among gay men using London gyms. *AIDS*, 15:1409-1415.

Elford, J., Bolding, G. & Sherr, L. (2001b), HIV optimism: Fact or fiction? *Focus*, 16:1-4.

Fleming, D.T. & Wasserheit, J.N. (1999), From epidemiological synergy to public health policy and practice: The contribution of other sexually transmitted diseases to sexual transmission of HIV infection. *Sexually Transmitted Infections*, 75:3-17.

Fleming, P.L., Byers, R.H., Sweeney, P.A., Daniels, D., Karon, J.M. & Janssen, R.S. (2002), *HIV Prevalence in the United States, 2000*. Paper presented at the 9th Conference on Retroviruses and Opportunistic Infections, Seattle, WA, February.

Frosch, D., Shoptaw, S., Huber, A., Rawson, R.A. & Ling, W. (1996), Sexual HIV risk among gay and bisexual male methamphetamine abusers. *J. Substance Abuse Treatment*, 13:483-486.

Gauthier, D.K. & Forsyth, C.J. (1999), Bareback sex, bug chasers, and the gift of death. *Deviant Behavior*, 20:85-100.

Gold, R. (1995), Why we need to rethink AIDS education for gay men. *AIDS Care*, 7 (Suppl 1):S11-S19.

Gold, R.S. & Skinner, M.J. (1996), Judging a book by its cover: Gay men's use of perceptible characteristics to infer antibody status. *International J. STD & AIDS*, 7:39-43.

Gold, R.S., Skinner, M.J. & Hinchy, J. (1999), Gay men's stereotypes about who is HIV infected: A further study. *International J. STD & AIDS*, 10:600-605.

Gold, R.S., Skinner, M.J. & Ross, M. (1994), Unprotected anal intercourse in HIV-infected and non-HIV-infected gay men. *J. Sex Research*, 31:59-77.

Goodroad, B.K., Kirksey, K.M. & Butensky, E. (2000), Bareback sex and gay men: An HIV prevention failure. *J. Association of Nurses in AIDS Care*, 11:29-36.

Halkitis, P.N., Parsons, J.T. & Stirratt, M.J. (2001), A double epidemic: Crystal methamphetamine drug use in relation to HIV transmission among gay men. *J. Homosexuality*, 41:17-35.

Halkitis, P.N., Parsons, J.T. & Wilton, L. (2003a), Barebacking among gay and bisexual men in New York City: Explanations for the emergence of intentional unsafe behavior. *Archives Sexual Behavior*, 32:351-357.

Halkitis, P.N., Parsons, J.T. & Wilton, L. (2003b), An exploratory study of contextual and situational factors related to methamphetamine use among gay and bisexual men in New York City. *J. Drug Issues*, 33:413-432.

Halkitis, P.N., Wilton, L., Parsons, J.T. & Hoff, C.C. (2004), Correlates of sexual risk-taking behavior among HIV-positive gay men in concordant primary partner relationships. *Psychology, Health, & Medicine*, 19: 99-113.

Halkitis, P.N., Wilton, L., Wolitski, R.J., Parsons, Hoff, J.T., & C. Bimbi, D. (2005), Barebacking identity amoung HIV-positive gay and bisexual men: Demographic, psychological, and behavior correlates. *AIDS*(Supp1): 527-535.

Hospers, H.J. & Kok, G. (1995), Determinants of safe and risk-taking sexual behavior among gay men: A review. *AIDS Education & Prevention*, 7:74-96.

International Collaboration on HIV Optimism (2003), HIV treatments optimism among gay men: An international perspective. *J. Acquired Immune Deficiency Syndromes & Human Retrovirology*, 32:545-550.

Jaffe, H.W. (2003), *HIV/AIDS in America Today*. Paper presented at the 2003 National HIV Prevention Conference, Atlanta, GA, July.

Janssen, R.S., Holtgrave, D.R., Valdiserri, R.O., Shepherd, M., Gayle, H.D. & DeCock, K.M. (2001), The serostatus approach to fighting the HIV epidemic: Prevention strategies for infected individuals. *American J. Public Health*, 91:1019-1024.

Kalichman, S.C. Nachimson, D., Cherry, C. & Williams, E. (1998), AIDS treatment advances and behavioral prevention setbacks: Preliminary assessment of reduced perceived threat of HIV-AIDS. *Health Psychology*, 17:546-550.

Kalichman, S.C., Rompa, D., Austin, J., Luke, W. & DiFonzo, K. (2001), Viral load, perceived infectivity, and unprotected intercourse. *J. Acquired Immune Deficiency Syndromes*, 28:303-305.

Kalichman, S.C., Weinhardt, L., Benotsch, E. & Cherry, C. (2002), Closing the digital divide in HIV/AIDS care: Development of a theory-based intervention to increase Internet access. *AIDS Care*, 14:523-537.

Katz, M.H., Schwarcz, S.K., Kellogg, T.A., Klausner, J.D., Dilley, J.W., Gibson, S. & McFarland, W. (2002), Impact of highly active retroviral treatment on HIV seroincidence among men who have sex with men: San Francisco. *American J. Public Health*, 92:388-394.

Kelly, J.A., Hoffmann, R.G., Rompa, D. & Gray, M. (1998), Protease inhibitor combination therapies and perceptions of gay men regarding AIDS severity and the need to maintain safer sex. *AIDS*, 12:F91-F95.

Kim, A.A., Kent, C., McFarland, W. & Klausner, J.D. (2001), Cruising on the Internet highway. *J. Acquired Immune Deficiency Syndromes*, 28:89-93.

Kippax, S. (2002), Negotiated safety agreements among gay men. In: *Beyond Condoms: Alternative Approaches to HIV Prevention*, ed. A. O'Leary. New York: Kluwer/Plenum Press, pp. 1-15.

Kippax, S. & Race, K. (2003), Sustaining safe practice: Twenty years on. *Social Science & Medicine*, 57:1-12.

Klausner, J.D., Wolf, W., Fischer-Ponce, L., Zolt, I. & Katz, M. (2000), Tracing a syphilis outbreak through cyberspace. *J. American Medical Association*, 284: 447-449.

MacKellar, D.A., Valleroy, L., Secura, G., Behel, S., Bingham, T., Shehen, D., LaLota, M., Celentano, D., Theiede, H., Koblin, B. & Torian, L. (2002), *Unrecognized HIV Infection, Risk Behavior, and Misperception of Risk Among Young Men Who Have Sex with Men–6 U.S. Cities, 1994-2000.* Poster presented at the XIV International Conference on AIDS, Barcelona, Spain, July.

Mansergh, G., Colfax, G.N., Marks, G., Rader, M., Guzman, R. & Buchbinder, S. (2001), The Circuit Party Men's Health Survey: Findings and implications for gay and bisexual men. *American J. Public Health,* 91:953-958.

Mansergh, G., Marks, G., Colfax, G.N., Guzman, R., Rader, M. & Buchbinder, S. (2002), "Barebacking" in a diverse sample of men who have sex with men. *AIDS,* 16:653-659.

Marks, G., Burris, S. & Peterman, T.A. (1999), Reducing sexual transmission of HIV from those who know they are infected: The need for personal and collective responsibility. *AIDS,* 13:297-306.

National Institute on Drug Abuse (1998), *NIDA Community Drug Alert Bulletin– Methamphetamine,* October.

Nimmons, D. & Folkman, S. (1999), Other-sensitive motivation for safer sex among gay men: Expanding paradigms for HIV prevention. *AIDS & Behavior,* 3:313-324.

O'Brien, T.R., Kedes, D., Ganem, D., Macrae, D.R., Rosenberg, P.S., Molden, J. & Goedert, J.J. (1999), Evidence of concurrent epidemics of human herpes virus 8 and human immunodeficiency virus type-1 in US homosexual men: Rates, risk factors, and relationship to Kaposi's Sarcoma. *J. Infectious Disease,* 180:1010-1017.

O'Leary, A., Purcell, D., Remien, R.H. & Gomez, C. (2003), Childhood sexual abuse and sexual transmission risk behaviour among HIV-positive men who have sex with men. *AIDS Care,* 15:17-26.

Odets, W. (1994), AIDS education and harm reduction for gay men: Psychological approaches for the 21st century. *AIDS & Public Policy Journal,* 9:1-15.

Ostrow, D.E., Fox, K.J., Chmiel, J.S., Silvestre, A., Visscher, B.R., Vanable, P. A., Jacobson, L.P. & Strathdee, S.A. (2002), Attitudes towards highly active antiretroviral therapy are associated with sexual risk taking among HIV-infected and uninfected homosexual men. *AIDS,* 16:775-780.

Purcell, D.W., Parsons, J.T., Halkitis, P.N., Mizuno, Y. & Woods, W.J. (2001), Substance use and sexual transmission risk behavior of HIV-positive men who have sex with men. *J. Substance Abuse,* 13:185-200.

Quinn, T.C., Wawer, M.J., Sewankambo, N., Serwadda, D., Li, C., Wabwire-Mangen, F., Meehan, M.O., Lutalo, T. & Gray, R.H. for the Rakai Project Study Group (2000), Viral load and heterosexual transmission of human immunodeficiency virus type 1. *New England Journal Medicine,* 342:921-929.

Rawson, R.A., Anglin, M.D., & Ling, W. (2002), Will the methamphetamine problem go away? *J. Addictive Diseases,* 21:5-19.

Remien, R.H., Carballo-Dieguez, A. & Wagner, G. (1995), Intimacy and sexual risk behaviour in serodiscordant male couples. *AIDS Care,* 7:429-438.

Reverson, T.A. & Schiaffino, K.M. (2000), Community-based health interventions. In: *Handbook of Community Psychology,* eds. J. Rappaport & E. Seidman. New York: Kluwer Academic/Plenum Publishers, pp. 471-493.

Rogers, S.M. & Turner, C. F. (1991), Male-male sexual contact in the USA: Findings from five sample surveys, 1970-1990. *J. Sex Research*, 28:491-519.

Romanelli, F., Smith, K.M. & Pomeroy, C. (2003), Use of club drugs by HIV-seropositive and HIV-seronegative gay and bisexual men. *Topics in HIV Medicine*, 11:25-32.

Rotello, G. (1997), *Sexual Ecology: AIDS and the Destiny of Gay Men.* New York: Dutton.

Rothenberg, R.B., Scarlett, M., del Rio, C., Reznik, D. & O'Daniels, C. (1998), Oral transmission of HIV. *AIDS*, 12:2095-2105.

Savage, D. (1999), Bucking the condomocracy. *Out Magazine*, p. 34, July.

Scarce, M. (1999), A ride on the wild side. *Poz*, February, Available at: http://www.poz.com/archive/february1999/inside/rideonthewild.html. Accessed July 14, 2003.

Schwartz, D. & Bailey, C. (2005), Between the sheets and between the ears: Sexual practices and risk beliefs. In: *HIV + Sex: The Psychological and Intrapersonal Dynamics of HIV-Seropositive Gay and Bisexual Men's Relationships*, eds. P.N. Halkitis, C. Gómez & R.J. Wolitski. Washington, DC: American Psychological Association.

Shilts, R. (1987), *And the Band Played On: Politics, People, and the AIDS Epidemic.* New York: St. Martin's Press.

Stall, R., Mills, TC, Williamson, J., Hart, T., Greenwood, G., Paul, J., Pollack, L., Binson, D., Osmond, D., & Catania, J.A. (2003), Association of co-occurring psychosocial health problems and increased vulnerability to HIV/AIDS among urban MSM. *American J. of Public Health*, 93: 939-942.

Stall, R., Paul, J.P., Greenwood, G., Pollack, L.M., Bein, E., Crosby, G.M., Mills, T.C., Binson, D., Coates, T.J. & Catania, J.A. (2001), Alcohol use, drug use and alcohol-related problems among men who have sex with men: The Urban Men's Health Study. *Addiction*, 96:1589-1601.

Stall, R. & Purcell, D.W. (2000), Intertwining epidemics: A review of research on substance use among men who have sex with men and its connection to the AIDS epidemic. *AIDS & Behavior*, 4:181-192.

Stall, R.D., Waldo, C.R., Ekstrand, M. & McFarland, W. (2000), The Gay 90s: A review of research in the 1990s on sexual behavior and HIV risk among men who have sex with men. *AIDS*, 14(Suppl 3):S101-S114.

Suarez, T. & Miller, J. (2001), Negotiating risks in context: A perspective on unprotected anal intercourse and barebacking among men who have sex with men–Where do we go from here? *Archives Sexual Behavior*, 30:287-300.

Sumartojo, E. (2000), Structural factors in HIV prevention: Concepts, examples, and implications for research. *AIDS*, 14(Suppl 1):S3-S10.

Tubiana, R., Ghosn, J., De-Sa, M., Wirden, M., Gautheret-Dejean, A., Bricaire, F. & Katlama, C. (2002), Warning: Antiretroviral treatment interruption could lead to an increased risk of HIV transmission. *AIDS*, 16:1083-1084.

Van de Ven, P., Kippax, S., Crawford, J., Rawstorne, P., Prestage, G., Grulich, A. & Murphy, D. (2002), In a minority of gay men, sexual risk practice indicates strategic positioning for perceived risk reduction rather than unbridled sex. *AIDS Care*, 14:471-480.

Vanable, P.A., Ostrow, D.G., McKirnan, D.J., Taywaditep, K.J. & Hope, B.A. (2000), Impact of combination therapies on HIV risk perceptions and sexual risk among

HIV-positive and HIV-negative gay and bisexual men. *Health Psychology*, 19: 134-145.

Weinhardt, L.S., Carey, M.P.,Johnson, B.T. & Bickham, N.L. (1999), Effects of HIV counseling and testing on sexual risk behavior: A meta-analytic review of published research, 1985-1997. *American J. Public Health*, 89.1397-1405.

Wiley, D.J., Visscher, B.R., Grosser, S., Hoover, D.R., Day, R., Gange, S., Chmiel, J.S., Mitsuyasu, R. & Detels, R. (2000), Evidence that anoreceptive intercourse with ejaculate exposure is associated with rapid CD4 loss. *AIDS*, 14:707-715.

Wilton, L. (2001), Perceived health risks and psychosocial factors as predictors of sexual risk-taking within HIV-positive gay male seroconcordant couples, *Dissertation Abstracts International*, 61 (7-B), 3867.

Wolitski, R.J., Bailey, C., O'Leary, A., Gómez, C.A., Parsons, J.T. & the Seropositive Urban Men's Study Group (2003), Self-perceived responsibility of HIV-seropositive men for preventing HIV transmission to sex partners. *AIDS & Behavior*, 7:363-372.

Wolitski, R.J. & Branson, B.M. (2002), "Gray area behaviors" and partner selection strategies: Working toward a comprehensive approach to reducing the sexual transmission of HIV. In: *Beyond Condoms: Alternative Approaches to HIV Prevention*, ed. A. O'Leary. New York: Kluwer/Plenum Press, pp. 173-198.

Wolitski, R.J., Janssen, R.S., Holtgrave, D.R. & Peterson, J.L. (2004), The public health response to the HIV epidemic in the United States. In: *AIDS and Other Manifestations of HIV Infection (4th ed.)*, ed. G. Wormser. San Diego: Academic Press/Elsevier Science, pp. 997-1012.

Wolitski, R.J., Mac Gowan, R.J., Higgins, D.L. & Jorgensen, C.M. (1997), The effects of HIV counseling and testing on risk-related practices and help-seeking behavior. *AIDS Education & Prevention*, 9 (Suppl. B):52-67.

Wolitski, R.J., Valdiserri, R.O., Denning, P.H. & Levine, W.C. (2001), Are we headed for a resurgence in the HIV epidemic among men who have sex with men? *American J. Public Health*, 91:883-888.

Yep, G.A., Lovaas, K.E. & Pagonis, A. V. (2002), The case of "riding bareback": Sexual practices and the paradoxes of identity in the era of AIDS. *J. Homosexuality*, 42(2):1-14.

What's in a Term?
How Gay and Bisexual Men
Understand Barebacking

Perry N. Halkitis, PhD
Leo Wilton, PhD
Paul Galatowitsch, PhD

SUMMARY. This study examines conceptual understandings, definitions, and practices of barebacking in a sample of 227 gay and bisexual men recruited from four gay venues in the New York Metropolitan
area. Findings demonstrated that 21% of the participants identified
as HIV-negative (HIV−) and 61.7% as HIV-positive (HIV+). While 90%
of the sample was familiar with the term "barebacking," differences
were noted in conceptual understandings and practices of barebacking between HIV+ and HIV− men. In particular, the findings suggest that these men were more likely to socialize and have sex with

---

Perry N. Halkitis is Associate Professor and Chair, Department of Applied
Psychology, New York University, and Director, Center for Health, Identity, Behavior,
and Prevention Studies (CHIBPS).

Leo Wilton is Assistant Professor, Departments of Human Development and Africana Studies, Binghamton University, State University of New York.

Paul Galatowitsch is affiliated with the Center for Health, Identity, Behavior, and Prevention Studies.

Address correspondence to: Perry N. Halkitis, PhD, New York University, 239
Greene Street, Suite 408, New York, NY 10003 (E-mail: pnh1@nyu.edu).

[Haworth co-indexing entry note]: "What's in a Term? How Gay and Bisexual Men Understand
Barebacking." Halkitis, Perry N., Leo Wilton, and Paul Galatowitsch. Co-published simultaneously in *Journal
of Gay & Lesbian Psychotherapy* (The Haworth Medical Press, an imprint of The Haworth Press, Inc.) Vol. 9,
No. 3/4, 2005, pp. 35-48; and: *Barebacking: Psychosocial and Public Health Approaches* (ed: Perry N. Halkitis,
Leo Wilton, and Jack Drescher) The Haworth Medical Press, an imprint of The Haworth Press, Inc., 2005,
pp. 35-48. Single or multiple copies of this article are available for a fee from The Haworth Document Delivery
Service [1-800-HAWORTH, 9:00 a.m. - 5:00 p.m. (EST). E-mail address: docdelivery@haworthpress.com].

doi:10.1300/J236v09n03_03   *35* seroconcordant partners and that these patterns of socialization may shape attitudes and practices about barebacking. *[Article copies available for a fee from The Haworth Document Delivery Service: 1-800-HAWORTH. E-mail address: <docdelivery@haworthpress.com> Website: <http://www.HaworthPress.com>* © 2005 by The Haworth Press, Inc. All rights reserved.]*

KEYWORDS. AIDS, anal sex, barebacking, bisexual, gay, HIV, homosexuality, men who have sex with men (MSM), oral sex, sexual practices, unsafe sex

INTRODUCTION

Twenty years after the initial diagnoses of HIV in the United States (U.S.), gay and bisexual men continue to engage in unsafe sexual behaviors (Halkitis et al., 2005; Kellogg, McFarland and Katz, 1999; Parsons et al., 2003; Wolitski et al., 2001). To this end, the rate of new HIV diagnoses among men-who-have-sex-with-men (MSM), who are primarily gay or bisexual identified, has increased by 14% between 1999 and 2001 (CDC, 2003). For HIV-negative (HIV−) men, initial infection with HIV and other sexually transmitted infections (STIs) are the most immediate consequence of unsafe transmission behaviors and are heightened by the potential for initial infection with medication resistant/untreatable HIV mutant variants (Boden et al., 1999). For HIV-positive (HIV+) men, unsafe sexual acts may place them at risk for "superinfection" (Schiltz and Sandfort, 2000), rapid loss of CD4 cells (Wiley et al., 2000), contracting other STIs that may lead to immune system deterioration (Bonell, Weatherburn and Hickson, 2000; Gibson, Pendo and Wohlfeiler, 1999), potential exposure to pathogens that may cause Kaposi's Sarcoma (O'Brien et al., 1999; Renwick et al., 1998), or co-infection with Hepatitis C (Flichman et al., 1999) that may compromise the efficacy of liver-burdensome antiretroviral regimens.

It is suggested that the practice of unprotected anal intercourse, the riskiest of HIV transmission-related behaviors (Vittinghoff et al., 1999), appears to have re-emerged strongly in the last several years, due in part to relapse from safer sex, but also to the increasingly popular behavioral phenomenon referred to as "barebacking" (Gauthier and Forsyth, 1999; Goodroad, Kirksey and Butensky, 2000; Halkitis and Parsons, 2003; Halkitis, Parsons and Wilton, 2003; Halkitis et al., 2004; Mansergh et al., 2002; Yep, Lovaas and Pagonis, 2002). Barebacking appears to have grown in the gay and bisexual male communities across the U.S. as evidenced by a handful of formative behavioral investigations, which have attempted to quantify this behavior (Carballo-Dieguez and Bauermeister, 2004; Halkitis and Parsons, 2003; Halkitis et al., 2003; Mansergh et al., 2002). While these quantitative data provide evidence that barebacking is an act of intention for unsafe anal intercourse, the data indicate the need for a further and deeper understanding of the behavior.

It is our belief that barebacking represents a very different type of sexual experience than those traditionally examined in HIV behavioral research, and that the construct of barebacking is poorly defined. Further, we assert that gay and bisexual men may use differing heuristics in understanding this behavior, and negotiating the sexual safety associated with it. Even among those published studies noted above, the behavioral research regarding barebacking remains limited with regard to the fact that there may be incongruence between "scientific" definitions of barebacking and the manner in which the behavior is understood at the community level.

To this end, the prevalence of barebacking among gay and bisexual men has continued to be an area of speculation since only four empirical investigations have been published with regard to this sexual behavior. More importantly, these studies have applied measures of barebacking with slightly differing definitions of the terms, and have used differing samples and recruitment strategies. Halkitis et al. (2003) estimate that 46% of a sample of HIV+ and HIV− MSM recruited in NYC-based community venues and who were familiar with the term reported bareback behavior when the term was used without any clarifying definition. In a study of HIV+ men recruited via the Internet from across the U.S., 84% reported barebacking in the three months prior to assessment (Halkitis and Parsons, 2003). However, in this case, the behavior was defined as being either insertive or receptive anal intercourse with any type of partner, and was assessed separately for partners of differing HIV serostatus. Mansergh et al. (2002) indicate that 14% of their sample recruited in San Francisco and familiar with the term barebacking reported this behavior when it was defined as "intentional anal sex without a condom with someone other than a primary partner." Further, the work of Carballo-Dieguez and Bauermesiter (2004) is based on a content analysis of Internet postings, thus not disentangling the meanings that these men had assigned to their postings.

Thus, we conducted a community-based cross-sectional study to assess definitions that gay and bisexual men ascribe to barebacking, specifically in how men relate this construct to actual behaviors and types of sexual partners. Our goal was to consider the extent to which there was consensus in the gay and bisexual community about what barebacking actually represents, as well as to gather further behavioral data on the frequency of this behavior.

METHOD

Participants

A total of 227 men completed the survey questionnaire. The participants were recruited actively through the distribution of brief intercept questionnaires at one of four venues in the New York Metropolitan area: 58.6% ($n = 133$) at a large gay/lesbian exposition, 17.2% ($n = 39$) on the street in a heavy populated gay neighborhood, 19.8% ($n = 45$) at a second such neighborhood, and 4.4% ($n = 10$) outside a Manhattan bar. Because the investigation sought to understand the meanings that gay and bisexual men ascribed to barebacking, individuals were eliminated whose sexual identities were not provided or who considered themselves heterosexual. This resulted in a final sample of 217 gay or bisexual men to consider in the present study. In terms of age, race, education level, and HIV serostatus, this final sample was equivalent to the original sample of 227 after eliminating those who did not indicate a gay or bisexual identity. A total of 17 hours across eight recruitment shifts were required to ascertain these participants.

On average, the participants were 39-years-old (SD = 9.17, Range = 20 to 66). In terms of race/ethnicity, 60.8% ($n = 138$) identified as White, 19.4% ($n = 44$) as African American, 13.2% ($n = 30$) as Latino, 3.5% ($n = 8$) as Asian/Pacific Islander, and 5.7% ($n = 13$) as some other race or of mixed race; two respondents failed to answer this question. The majority of the men identified as gay (86.3%, $n = 196$), followed by bisexual (8.4%, $n = 19$), and "on the downlow" (0.9%, $n = 2$). The remainder either identified as heterosexual, "other," or failed to respond to this question. In terms of HIV status, 21.1% ($n = 48$) reported that they were HIV+ and 140 (61.7%) HIV– ; 1.8% ($n = 4$) were not tested but suspected that they were HIV+, and 9.3% ($n = 21$) had not tested but suspected they were HIV– . Fourteen individuals did not respond to this item. Finally, in terms of educational background, 62.1% ($n = 141$)

reported a college or higher level degree and 32.5% (*n* = 74) reported some college or less, with 12 individuals failing to answer this question.

Measures

The survey was a two-sided, tri-fold questionnaire that required an average of five minutes to complete. In addition to sociodemographic questions, the survey contained the following measures:

Familiarity with Term Barebacking. An initial item posed the statement "I am familiar with the term barebacking." Those who responded "Yes" were then instructed to provide a definition for the term. Those who were not familiar with the term were instructed to skip the proceeding questions regarding barebacking and simply provided demographic information.

Characteristics of Barebacking. A set of five stand-alone items assessed the participants' perceived characteristics of barebackers and barebacking. The first question sought to determine the role of intention in barebacking and stated, "According to me, a guy would be barebacking if he had unprotected anal sex and did not use a condom if (1) he had never intended to use a condom; (2) he intended to use a condom but in the heat of the moment did not; or (3) both of the above." Second, participants were asked if a barebacker was sexually "a top," "a bottom," or "either." Third, participants were asked about their perception of the HIV serostatus of barebackers (if barebackers tended to be HIV+, HIV−, HIV status unknown, or any of the above). In terms of partners, subjects were asked if barebacking is a term that men applied to lovers/partners, casual partners, fuck buddies, sex workers, or all of the above. And finally, "According to me, barebacking is a term that applies to oral sex."

Barebacking Behavior. One individual item assessed barebacking behavior: "Based on your definition of barebacking, do you bareback?" Those who indicated that they did bareback were asked to indicate their sexual roles with partners of varying HIV serostatus. In this regard, three separate questions were asked of the men regarding when they bareback with men who were HIV+, HIV−, or HIV status unknown if they were (1) always a top, (2) usually a top, (3) sometimes a top and sometimes a bottom, (4) usually a bottom, or (5) always a bottom. A final response choice indicated that the participant did not bareback with that serostatus partner type.

RESULTS

Characteristics of Barebacking

The results of our analyses are based on the 217 men who had indicated a sexual identity of gay or bisexual. In terms of familiarity with the term barebacking, the majority of the participants were familiar with the term (89.9%, n = 195). There were no differences in age, race/ethnicity, HIV serostatus, educational background, or recruitment venue between those respondents familiar and unfamiliar with the term.

Of the 195 participants familiar with the term, there was an overwhelming sentiment that barebacking referred to both sexual situations in which there was never an intent to use a condom as well as in situations of relapse in condom use during unprotected sex (i.e., "in the heat of the moment"). Overall, 73.8% (n = 144) of the men familiar with the term barebacking indicated that it could be properly applied to either situation. Only 3.1% (n = 6) suggested that barebacking was a term related solely to a relapse-related episode, and 18.5% (n = 36) to unsafe episodes that were intended. Nine participants failed to respond or were unsure. No differences were noted across any of the demographic factors.

We also coded the written responses that the participants provided when asked to indicate their definitions of the term barebacking. Of those familiar with the term, 44.1% (n = 86) provided a definition that indicated the behavior referred to a situation where there was anal sex and in which there was no use of a condom. These definitions included responses such as "anal sex without a condom," "anal intercourse without a condom," "anal penetration without a rubber," "fucking without a condom," and "unprotected fucking." A smaller group (25.1%, n = 49) suggested a definition that referred to sex in general (not specifically anal sex) without a condom. Examples of these definitions included "sex without a condom," "condomless sex," and "unprotected sex." Overall, 74.4% indicated a definition that included sex in general or anal sex. Of the remaining 50 individuals, 22 provided a definition that included only a statement about the absence of condom use but no reference to sex, 15 provided no definition, and 7 provided a value judgment of the behavior rather than a definition. Included among the latter were statements such as "being stupid," "being a suicidal idiot and killing others, and "a blatant disregard for safety." It should be noted that only one individual included the construct of intent in his definition, "anal sex, no condom, on purpose."

In terms of HIV serostatus and sexual roles of barebackers, 91.8% (n = 179) indicated that a barebacker could be "top" or "bottom," and 66.2% (n = 129) indicated that barebackers could be of any HIV serostatus. Table 1 provides a description of the types of partners that the men associated with barebacking. Participants were permitted to check more than one response. As is shown, the majority of the participants (89.7%, n = 175) indicated that sex could be considered bareback when the act involved a lover/partner, casual partner, fuck buddy, or sex worker, while 6.2% reported that barebacking is a term that only can be applied to sexual episodes with casual partners and/or fuck buddies.

The responses were less definitive with regard to the term barebacking being applied to oral sex. While 65.1% (n = 127) indicated that the term was not applicable to oral sex, 15.4% (n = 36) indicated that it was applicable; more importantly, 18.5% (n = 36) were unsure if the term was applicable to oral sex. Furthermore, participants who included the term "anal sex" in their definitions of barebacking were less likely, as compared to those who used a non-specified type of sex in their definitions, to indicate that barebacking referred to oral sex and were less likely to be unsure if the term referred to barebacking ($\chi^2(2) = 11.91$, $p < .01$). Specifically, while only 4.5% of those who defined barebacking in terms of anal sex believed that oral sex was also barebacking, 20.0% of those who defined the term as a non-specified type of sex believed barebacking included oral sex. Further, while only 13.5% of those who defined barebacking as anal sex were unsure if the term referred to oral sex, 21.8% of those who did not specify the type of

TABLE 1. Frequencies of Types of Partners Associated with Barebacking

Partner Type	n	%
Casual Partner only	3	1.5%
Fuck Buddy only	5	2.6%
Casual Partner or Fuck Buddy	4	2.1%
Main Partner only	7	3.6%
Sex Worker only	0	0.0%
Any type	175	89.7%
Missing	1	< 1%
TOTAL	195	

sex associated with barebacking in their definitions were unsure if the term included oral sex behaviors.

Barebacking Behavior

With regard to the practice of barebacking, 34.9% (n = 68) indicated that they engaged in this behavior. However, this was reported at differential rates across participant HIV serostatus ($\chi^2(1)$ = 6.10, p = .01). Specifically, while 50% of the men who reported being HIV+ or believed they were HIV+ practiced barebacking, only 29.9% of those who reported being HIV− or believed that they were HIV− practiced this behavior. Thus, HIV+ men were about two times more likely to practice barebacking than HIV− men (OR = 2.34, 95% CI 1.18, 4.64). No differences in self-reported barebacking were indicated across race/ethnicity or sexual identity.

Of the 68 men who reported that they practiced barebacking, 41 HIV− men and 23 HIV+ men reported their sexual roles when barebacking with partners who were HIV+, HIV− , or HIV status unknown. These are shown in Table 2, and indicate differential rates between HIV+ and HIV− in terms of the sexual roles in which they engage when they bareback with partners of varying HIV serostatus. The HIV+ participants reported proportionally equal rates of being a top, bottom, either, or not barebacking with all three types of partners. Thus, within each type of serostatus partner, HIV+ men engaged equally in each of the four sexual roles when they barebacked. However, among HIV− men, there were significant differences in the type of sexual role in which they engaged based on the serostatus of their partners. With regard to their HIV+ partners, HIV− men reported a greater likelihood not to engage in barebacking behavior ($\chi^2(2)$ = 45.71, p < .001). Specifically, 82.8% (n = 34) of the 41 HIV− men reported no barebacking with HIV+ partners. With their seroconcordant HIV− partners, they were more likely to engage in insertive anal intercourse as compared to all other sexual roles, although they also reported receptive anal intercourse and being either a top or bottom in these bareback experiences ($\chi^2(3)$ = 12.37, p < .01). With their status unknown partners, there was a marginal tendency to take on the role of top when barebacking ($\chi^2(3)$ = 7.29, p = .06).

TABLE 2. Barebacking Sexual Roles

	Top or Usually Top	Bottom or Usually Bottom	Top or Bottom	No Bareback	p*
HIV – Men (n = 41)					
HIV – Partners	39.0%	26.9%	31.7%	2.4%	< .01
HIV + Partners	12.2%	0.0%	4.9%	82.8%	< .001
HIV UK Partners	41.5%	14.6%	17.1%	26.8%	.06
HIV + Men (n = 23)					
HIV – Partners	12.0%	21.7%	47.8%	17.4%	.08
HIV + Partners	17.4%	21.7%	43.5%	17.4%	.23
HIV UK Partners	13.0%	34.8%	43.5%	26.1%	.17

* χ^2 (3)

DISCUSSION

This community-based study represents an initial attempt in elucidating the meanings that gay and bisexual men ascribe to barebacking. Our results suggest that barebacking is a term with which most gay and bisexual men are familiar but that it is not consistently defined. For some of the participants, barebacking is any form of unprotected sex; for others, barebacking refers only to unprotected anal sex even if unintended or intentional acts of unprotected anal intercourse. The majority of men in this study defined barebacking simply as anal intercourse without a condom, even if unintended. Another notable finding is the small number of men who associated unprotected oral sex with the term.

A smaller subset of men indicated that barebacking is a behavior that they practice, although the behavior was more common among HIV + men, particularly with their HIV + partners. These behavioral data regarding the practice of barebacking are comparable, although not identical to those in other published studies (Halkitis and Parsons, 2003; Halkitis et al., 2004; Mansergh et al., 2002). Variations in measurement procedures, sampling techniques, and definitions of the term across the studies are the likely explanation for these slight differences. The lack of consistency in defining barebacking among researchers also appears to be reflective of the varied understandings of barebacking in the larger gay community. However, barebacking practices did not significantly differ by race/ethnicity, indicating that in our sample of gay men, the practice is one that transgresses race and culture.

We also found significant differences between how HIV+ and HIV− men define and practice "barebacking." In our sample, HIV− men overwhelmingly indicate that barebacking, regardless of intention, is an act that HIV− men engage in with other HIV− men. Also, HIV− men reported that "barebackers" were more likely to be the insertive partner in unprotected anal sex. By contrast, HIV+ men reported that "barebackers" included both HIV + and HIV − men and that "barebackers" could be either insertive or receptive partners. This latter finding is consistent with patterns that have emerged in other studies of barebacking (Halkitis et al., 2004) and suggest a type of harm reduction approach to the behavior on the part of HIV− men. Further, 89% (*n* = 175) of the respondents reported that the partners of barebackers could be of any type, such as a "casual partner," "fuck buddy," "lover," or "sex worker." The remaining respondents specified a barebacker's partner type in one of the aforementioned categories.

These systematic differences in the conceptual understandings and practices of "barebacking" suggest that HIV+ and HIV− men have self-separated into seroconcordant social networks and that these social relationships are shaping the two groups' views of barebacking in different ways. The differing assumptions underlying barebacking that HIV+ and HIV− men hold may explain some of the misunderstandings that can lead HIV− men to assume, without discussing the matter, that their sexual partner is also HIV− and HIV+ men to assume that their sexual partner is HIV+. Further, the data also suggest that HIV− and HIV+ men employ different cognitive strategies to assist them in their decision not to use condoms. The success of these different cognitive strategies at preventing seroconversions or the extent to which they result in additional seroconversions cannot be known from this data. Nonetheless, these findings do point to the importance of considering this dynamic more thoroughly in HIV prevention messages.

Limitations

One of the major limitations of this formative behavioral investigation is the generalizability of the study's findings. The study's sample included only respondents in New York City and comprised a self-selected sample. However, the recruitment techniques that were employed, by gathering data at a variety of venues, helped to compensate for this matter. In addition, the demographic diversity of the sample is an indication that the data were collected from a more diverse sample of MSM that might not have been attained from data collection at one location or at one point in time.

As is the case with any questionnaire data, the self-reported indices may be undermined by the sensitive nature of the data being collected. To this end, the impact of socially desirable responses may have yielded behavioral indices which are underestimates of the practice of barebacking within the MSM community. However, we believe the issue of social desirability was minimized because our survey incorporated non-judgmental language in addition to our research team holding strong relationships and a level of trust with members of the MSM community.

Further, the nature of data collection, which included the completion of surveys in community and public settings, prevented us from gathering more in-depth and complex data. To this end, these findings must be viewed as information gathered from a brief intercept survey and should be considered a "snapshot" of the understanding and practice of the barebacking phenomenon rather than a large-scale systematic examination of the behavior. We believe that the barebacking phenomenon is complex, and that barebacking as a behavior and barebacking as an identity represent two very distinct polarities. To this end, our data suggest these differing aspects of barebacking and future investigations should seek to gather information that attempts to disentangle these elements.

Conclusions

Community-level interventions aimed at reducing the health risks among gay and bisexual men associated with barebacking should, as Wolitski (2005) points out, include the "involvement and support of community members and be culturally and ethnically diverse. Such efforts are less likely to be perceived as criticisms of the lifestyles of gay and bisexual men than would prevention programs coming from outside the community." Further, community-level interventions should also stress the downsides of HIV infection, side effects of HIV medications, long-term consequences of HIV, medication resistant HIV and so forth. Reminders of the deleterious effects of HIV infections may motivate clients to maintain increased awareness about becoming infected or infecting other potential partners.

Individual-level interventions may want to help both HIV+ and HIV− gay and bisexual men explore more critically their risk-reduction strategies. The strategies developed by Motivational Interviewing (MI) provide promising tools in that regard as Parsons (2005) describes in this volume. With HIV− men, for example, (1) therapists can help their clients realize that HIV+ and HIV− men may hold very different assumptions about barebacking and these differences can lead to miscommunications and misunderstandings about a partner's HIV status putting one or both partners at increased health risks; (2) HIV− men may report that they try to reduce their HIV transmission risk by asking partners their HIV status, therapists and counselors should point out that the majority of persons who test HIV+ mistakenly believed they were HIV− (Wolitski, 2005); (3) HIV− men may report that if an HIV+ partner reports having an undetectable viral load, the therapist can help their client understand that HIV is still transmissible and more likely to transmit a medication-resistant strain of HIV should infection occur. Assisting clients to critically evaluate their harm-reduction strategies combined with a therapeutic approach suggested by Nimmons and Folkman (1999) that emphasize how acquiring an HIV infection would affect a client's family, friends and future sexual partners and that avoiding HIV infection would also uphold personal and ethical values at safeguarding individual and community health. Interventions aimed at HIV+ men could use a similar strategy to educate men about the importance of protecting sex partners, and a desire to uphold personal ethical values.

Within this context, therapists must also consider the differential meanings that might be held by gay and bisexual men who bareback as compared to those who embrace a "barebacking identity," particularly as related to the experiences of HIV− as compared to HIV+ men (Halkitis et al., 2004). In all likelihood, the practice of these behaviors and the formation of these identities appear to evolve along differing developmental trajectories depending on the circumstances and contexts of each individual's life. To this end, the practice of unprotected anal intercourse, regardless of whether it is labeled barebacking or not, must be further considered in light of numerous other aspects of a person's life including culture, mental health, and drug-using behaviors. A holistic approach to understanding why some men bareback, why some men identify as barebackers and practice this behavior, and why some men reject this conception in its entirety is rooted in the life history of each individual that leads them to this place and time in which barebacking poses a threat to our community at large.

REFERENCES

Boden, D., Hurley, A., Zhang, L., Cao, Y., Guo, Y., Jones, E. et al. (1999), HIV− 1 drug resistance in newly infected individuals. *J. American Medical Association*, 282:1135-1141.

Bonnel, C., Weatherburn, P. & Hickson, F. (2000), Sexually transmitted infection as a risk factor for homosexual HIV transmission: A systematic review of epidemiological studies. *International J. STD & AIDS*, 11:697-700.

Carballo-Dieguez, A. & Bauermeister, J. (2004), "Barebacking": Intentional condomless anal sex in HIV− risk contexts: Reasons for and against it. *J. Homosexuality, 47:* 1-16.

Centers for Disease Control & Prevention (2003, November 28). Increases in HIV diagnoses–29 states, 1999-2003. *MMWR*, 52:1145-1148.

Flichman, D., Cello, J., Castano, G., Campos, R. & Sookoian, S. (1999), In vivo regulation of HIV replication after hepatitis superinfection. *Medicina*, 59:364-366.

Gauthier, D.K. & Forsyth, C.J. (1999), Bareback sex, bug chasers, and the gift of death. *Deviant Behavior*, 20:85-100.

Gibson, P., Pendo, M. & Wohlfeiler, D. (1999), Risk, HIV, and STD prevention. *Focus: A Guide to AIDS Research and Counseling*, 14:1-5.

Goodroad, B.K., Kirksey, K.M. & Butensky, E. (2000), Bareback sex and gay men: An HIV prevention failure. *J. Association of Nurses in AIDS Care*, 11:29-36.

Halkitis, P.N. & Parsons, J.T. (2003), Intentional unsafe sex (barebacking) among men who meet sexual partners on the Internet. *AIDS Care*, 15:367-378.

Halkitis, P.N., Parsons, J.T. & Wilton. L. (2003), Barebacking among gay and bisexual men in New York City: Explanations for the emergence of intentional unsafe behavior. *Archives Sexual Behavior*, 32:351-358.

Halkitis, P.N., Wilton, L., Parsons, J.T. & Hoff, C. (2004), Correlates of sexual risk-taking behavior among HIV seropositive gay men in seroconcordant primary partner relationships. *Psychology, Health, & Medicine*, 9:99-113.

Halkitis, P.N., Wilton, L., Wolitski, R.J., Parsons, J.T , Hoff, C. & Bimbi, D. (2005), Barebacking identity among HIV-positive gay and bisexual men: Demographic, psychological, and behavior correlates. *AIDS*(Suppl): 527-535.

Kellogg, T., McFarland, W. & Katz, M. (1999), Recent increase in HIV seroconversions among repeat anonymous testers in San Francisco. *AIDS*, 13:2303-2304.

Mansergh, G., Marks, G., Colfax, G., Guzman, R., Rader, M. & Buchbinder, S. (2002), Barebacking in a diverse sample of men who have sex with men. *AIDS*, 16:653-659.

Nimmons, D. & Folkman, S. (1999), Other-sensitive motivation for safer sex among gay men: Expanding paradigms for HIV prevention. *AIDS & Behavior*, 3:313-324.

O'Brien, T.R., Kedes, D., Ganem, D., Macrae, D., Rosenberg, P., Molden, J. et al. (1999), Evidence of concurrent epidemics of human herpesvirus 8 and human immunodeficiency virus type 1 in US homosexual men: Rates, risk factors, and relationship to Kaposi's Sarcoma. *J. Infectious Diseases*, 180:1010-1017.

Parsons, J.T. (2005), Motivating the unmotivated: A treatment model for barebackers. *J. Gay & Lesbian Psychotherapy*, 9(3/4): 129-148.

Parsons, J.T., Halkitis, P.N., Wolitski, R.J., Gomez, C.A. & the Seropositive Urban Men's Study Team (2003), Correlates of sexual risk behaviors among HIV+ men who have sex with men. *AIDS Education & Prevention*, 15:383-400.

Renwick, N., Halby, T., Weverling, G., Dukers, N., Simpson, G.R., Coutinho, R.A. et al. (1998), Seroconversion for human herpes virus 8 during HIV infection is highly predictive of Kaposi's sarcoma. *AIDS*, 12:2481-2488.

Schiltz, M.A., & Sandfort, T.G.M. (2000), HIV-positive people, risk, and sexual behaviours. *Social Science & Medicine*, 50:1571-1588.

Vittinghoff, E., Douglas, J., Judson, F., McKirnan, D., MacQueen, K. & Buchbinger, S.P. (1999), Per-contact risk of human immunodeficiency virus transmission between male sexual partners. *American J. Epidemiology*, 150:1-6.

Wiley, D.J., Visscher, B.R., Grosser S., Hoowever, D.R., Day, R., Gange, S. et al. (2000), Evidence that anoreceptive intercourse with ejaculate exposure is associated with rapid CD4 loss. *AIDS*, 14:707-715.

Wolitski, R.J. (2005), The emergence of barebacking among gay and bisexual men in the United States: A public health perspective. *J. Gay & Lesbian Psychotherapy*, 9(3/4):9-134.

Wolitski, R.J., Valdisserri, R.O., Denning, P.H. & Levine, W.C. (2001), Are we headed for a resurgence in the HIV epidemic among men who have sex with men? *American J. Public Health*, 91:883-888.

Yep, G.A., Lovaas, K.E. & Pagonis, A.V. (2002), The case of "riding bareback": Sexual practices and the paradoxes of identity in the era of AIDS. *J. Homosexuality*, 42:1-14.

An Exploratory Study of Barebacking, Club Drug Use, and Meanings of Sex in Black and Latino Gay and Bisexual Men in the Age of AIDS

Leo Wilton, PhD
Perry N. Halkitis, PhD
Gary English
Michael Roberson

SUMMARY. Current epidemiological trends demonstrate that Black and Latino men-who-have-sex-with-men (MSM) have increasingly disproportionate rates of HIV. The emergence of barebacking (intentional

Leo Wilton is Assistant Professor of Human Development and Africana Studies, Binghamton University, State University of New York.

Perry N. Halkitis is Associate Professor and Chair, Department of Applied Psychology, New York University, and Director, Center for Health, Identity, Behavior, and Prevention Studies (CHIBPS).

Gary English is Executive Director, and Michael Roberson is Director of Services, People of Color in Crisis (POCC), 468 Bergen Street, Brooklyn, NY 11217.

Address correspondence to: Leo Wilton, PhD, Binghamton University, School of Education and Human Development, P.O. Box 6000, Binghamton, NY 13902 (E-mail: lwilton@binghamton.edu).

This study was funded by the National Institute on Drug Abuse (Contact #13798), Halkitis (PI).

[Haworth co-indexing entry note]: "An Exploratory Study of Barebacking, Club Drug Use, and Meanings of Sex in Black and Latino Gay and Bisexual Men in the Age of AIDS." Wilton, Leo et al. Co-published simultaneously in *Journal of Gay & Lesbian Psychotherapy* (The Haworth Medical Press, an imprint of The Haworth Press, Inc.) Vol. 9, No. 3/4, 2005, pp. 49-72; and: *Barebacking: Psychosocial and Public Health Approaches* (ed: Perry N. Halkitis, Leo Wilton, and Jack Drescher) The Haworth Medical Press, an imprint of The Haworth Press, Inc., 2005, pp. 49-72. Single or multiple copies of this article are available for a fee from The Haworth Document Delivery Service [1-800-HAWORTH, 9:00 a.m. - 5:00 p.m. (EST). E-mail address: docdelivery@haworthpress.com].

unprotected anal intercourse) and club drug use (cocaine, methamphetamine, GHB, ecstasy, ketamine) have posed a significant public health threat for MSM. This formative, behavioral multi-method investigation aims to examine barebacking, club drug use, and meanings of sex in Black and Latino gay and bisexual (BLGB) men. The data were drawn from the baseline assessment of a larger-scale longitudinal investigation (N = 450) of club drug use in gay and bisexual men from the New York Metropolitan area recruited from mainstream gay venues, AIDS service organizations, and public/commercial sex environments. Findings demonstrated that Black and Latino men were more likely to report an HIV-positive serostatus and identify as bisexual. Significant racial/ethnic differences were demonstrated in the use of club drugs. HIV-positive men reported significantly more frequent barebacking with HIV-positive partners. Latino men of HIV unknown status perceived greater benefits of barebacking. The qualitative data suggested specific cultural and phenomenological meanings ascribed to the act of bareback sex, club drug use, and the intersection of these behaviors. *[Article copies available for a fee from The Haworth Document Delivery Service: 1-800-HAWORTH. E-mail address: <docdelivery@haworthpress.com> Website: <http://www.HaworthPress.com> © 2005 by The Haworth Press, Inc. All rights reserved.]*

KEYWORDS. African-American, AIDS, Black men, barebacking, bisexual men, club drugs, cocaine, drug use, ecstasy, gay men, GHB, HIV, homosexuality, ketamine, Latino men, men-who-have-sex-with-men, methamphetamine, sexual behavior, unprotected anal intercourse, unsafe sex

Since the onset of the AIDS epidemic, epidemiological data in the United States (U.S.) has demonstrated that men-who-have-sex-with-men (MSM) continue to engage in risk-taking behaviors with their sexual partners (CDC, 2004a; Chen et al., 2002; Halkitis et al., 2004; Wilton, 2001). These trends have resulted in an accelerated increase in the rate of HIV seroconversions, especially for Black and Latino MSM (CDC, 2002; Koblin et al., 2000; Mays, Cochran and Zamudio, 2004; Peterson and Carballo-Dieguez, 2000). In the Young Men's Survey, among 3,492 MSM (15-22) surveyed in seven cities across the U.S., seroprevalence rates were higher among Blacks (18.4%) and Latinos (8.8%) as compared to Whites (3.1%) (Valleroy et al., 2000). In the Young Men's Survey Phase II, among 2,942 men (23-29), HIV seroprevalence rates were significantly higher among Blacks (32% overall) and Latinos (14% overall) than Whites (7% overall) (CDC, 2001). With increases in the transmission of STDs, including HIV, some researchers have viewed a resurgence of the AIDS epidemic (Wolitski et al., 2001).

The emergence of barebacking has been situated within the broader context of increasing rates of HIV infection. Barebacking has been conceptualized as intentional unprotected anal intercourse (UAI), thus differentiating it from relapse from safer sex behavioral norms (Mansergh et al., 2002). Yet, a scarcity of scientific research has studied barebacking in MSM, particularly as related to Black and Latino gay and bisexual (BLGB) men. To date, there have been two published empirical studies that have examined racial/ethnic differences in relation to barebacking. In the first study, Mansergh et al. (2002) demonstrated that Black and Latino men, as compared to White men, reported less familiarity with the term barebacking, with no significant racial/ethnic differences related to the prevalence of barebacking. Second, Halkitis et al. (2005) found that 20.4% of Black and 22.4% of Latino men, as compared to 33.1% of White men, identified as barebackers; 2.7% of Other or Mixed Race men identified with this term. Further, the findings showed that while only 7.6% of White men were not familiar with the term, 25.0% of Black men, 21.4% of Latino men, and 14.3% of Other or Mixed Race men were not familiar with the term, inferring some differential use of the term across race/ethnicity.

Connected to the barebacking phenomena, research findings have substantiated the link between recreational drug use and sexual risk behavior, thus placing MSM at increased risk for HIV seroconversion (Clatts, 2004; Colfax et al., 2004; Diaz, Heckert and Sanchez, 2004; Fuller et al., 2004; Greenwood et al., 2001) due to the practice of UAI (Wilton, 2001). The use of recreational drugs has been described as having an important impact on many gay men's identities (Knox et al., 1999), and gay-identified venues serve as contexts in which drug use is nested within gay socialization (McKirnan et al., 1996). Further, some researchers have suggested that HIV prevention research examine the complexities and synergistic interactions of HIV and substance use as overlapping epidemics (Stall and Purcell, 2000). While gay men tend to identify substance use as a major cause of unprotected sex, substance-using gay men report unprotected insertive anal intercourse (UIAI) and unprotected receptive anal intercourse (URAI) at the rates of 21% and 23% respectively, with 32% indicating UIAI and/or URAI (Dolezal et al., 1997).

The increasing prevalence of a specific set of drugs, known colloquially as "club drugs" (i.e., cocaine, GHB, ketamine, methamphetamine, and MDMA or ecstasy; see McDowell, 2000) because of their association with gay dance clubs and other venues (sex clubs, bathhouses, bars) pose an immediate public health threat for BLGB men in terms of HIV risk behavior. Recent studies (Halkitis et al., 2005; Halkitis, Parsons and Wilton, 2003a; Parsons and Halkitis, 2002; Stall et al., 2001) of racially/ethnically diverse community based samples of HIV-positive and HIV-negative MSM have demonstrated the increasing prevalence of club drug use, suggesting that drug using behaviors in this population may permeate race/ethnicity, HIV serostatus, and sexual orientation (Carballo-Dieguez and Dolezal, 1996).

For example, Halkitis et al. (2005) found that barebackers, as compared to non-barebackers, were more likely to report the use of amphetamines, barbiturates, cocaine, ecstasy, ketamine, marijuana, inhalant nitrates, GHB, and methamphetamine as well as injecting drugs including amphetamine and methamphetamine within the three months prior to assessment. These club drugs influence the sexual behaviors of users because they are used in environments in which sex is the primary objective of participation (Bochow, 1998), demonstrating the increased relationship between club drug use and HIV transmission (Chesney, Barrett and Stall, 1998). Further, the use of club drugs presents adverse health risks including cardiovascular, neurological, and respiratory effects, as well as psychotic behavior, violence, and death (Klein and Kramer, 2004; Romanelli and Smith, 2004).

To better understand barebacking, club drug use, and meanings of sex in a community based sample of BLGB men, the researchers have undertaken an exploratory investigation that incorporates both quantitative and qualitative methodologies. We employ a multi-method methodological approach (Creswell, 2003) to understand the contextual interrelationships within a non-treatment seeking and community-based sample of men. Specifically, we examine major salient descriptive findings related to sociodemographic, barebacking, club drug use, and sexual behavior characteristics. Further, we explore the contextual factors associated with these factors based on the qualitative narratives of BLGB men. This approach to understanding AIDS-related behaviors, as part of formative research designed to inform interventions, has been recommended (Zeller, 1993).

METHOD

Participants and Procedure

The data described here were collected as part of a formative behavioral research investigation (Club Drug Use and Men's Health: A Community Study), which was funded by the National Institute of Drug Abuse (NIDA). The primary objective of this longitudinal study was to assess individual differences and changes in club drug use and develop drug-using trajectories among 450 gay and bisexual men in New York City over the course of one year, and to relate these trajectories to sexual risk-taking. Participants were assessed at four points in this longitudinal design: Baseline, 4-Month, 8-Month, and 12-Month. Participants received $30 at Baseline, $35 at 4-Month, $40 at 8-Month, and $50 at 12-Month assessments for participation in the study.

The primary criteria for inclusion in the study were that participants: (1) self-identified as gay or bisexual, biologically male, and at least 18 years of age; (2) reported at least six occasions in the use of a club drug in the year prior to screening (club drugs were identified as one of the following: cocaine, GHB, ketamine, MDMA, methamphetamine); one of these occasions must have been in the last quarter of that previous year; and (3) indicated the use of at least one incident in which a club drug was used in combination with a sexual episode in the year prior to assessment.

The researchers employed a targeted, community-based sampling strategy for research studies with MSM (Watters and Biernacki, 1989). A targeted sampling strategy aims to "obtain systematic information when true random sampling is not feasible and when convenience sampling is not rigorous enough to meet the assumptions of the research design" (Watters and Biernacki, 1989, p. 420). In the present investigation, targeted sampling provided a more culturally competent and relevant approach than convenience sampling (Metsch et al., 1998), and has been used in HIV prevention studies in order to minimize selection bias (Deren et al., 1998; Halkitis et al., 2004). By incorporating this approach, participants were recruited from mainstream gay venues, AIDS service organizations, and public/commercial sex environments through both active and passive recruitment strategies. Respondents interested in the study called a toll-free telephone number in order to be screened for eligibility.

Eligible participants were scheduled for a baseline assessment. After obtaining informed consent, participants completed a semi-structured interview including a Critical Incident Measure (CIM) (Ross et al., 1992) as a part of the Baseline Qualitative Protocol for approximately one-hour to assess contextual factors associated with club drug use and sexual risk-taking behaviors, including barebacking. Participants were then administered quantitative measures via the ACASI (Audio Computer Assisted Self Interviewing) system, a computer-based technology where participants listened to the survey questions through headphones and entered responses into a computer.

Following this procedure, the researchers conducted HIV confirmatory testing for participants reporting an HIV-negative or unknown status through the use of Orasure, the oral test of HIV antibodies, in order to ensure the accuracy of self-reported HIV status (Vargo et al., 2004). Participants who reported being HIV-positive were asked to provide verification of their HIV status. The Orasure procedure was administered via pre- and post-test counseling guidelines mandated by the New York State AIDS Institute as outlined by the New York State HIV Confidentiality Law. Besides providing accurate information about HIV status, the inclusion of HIV testing provided an ethical responsibility to participants who might not otherwise test for HIV.

Quantitative Measures

Sociodemographic Characteristics. Participants were asked to indicate their race/ethnicity, age, gender, sexual orientation, HIV status, educational background, current employment status, and total personal income during the last year.

Club Drug Use. Participants were asked to provide the frequency of club drug use (crystal methamphetamine, cocaine, ketamine, GHB, ecstasy) for a period of four months prior to assessment based on a 5-point, Likert scale (0 = *Never*, 1 = *Less Than Once a Month*, 2 = *Once to Two Times a Month*, 3 = *One to Two Times a Week*, 4 = *More Than Twice a Week*). For the purposes of the analyses, club drug use was categorized as non-use (never), binge use (less than once a month to 1-2 times a week), and chronic use (more than twice a week).

Barebacking Behaviors. Participants were asked to indicate whether or not they had engaged in bareback sex (intentional insertive and/or receptive anal intercourse) with a non-primary partner while high on club drugs in the four months prior to assessment. Participants responded to each set of questions separately by non-primary partner serostatus (HIV-positive, HIV-negative, and HIV unknown). For the purposes of the analyses, bareback behavior was collapsed across sexual role (insertive and receptive) and ejaculation (ejaculate transferred or ejaculate not transferred between sexual partners).

Benefits of Barebacking Scale (BOBS). The BOBS is a 9-item, 5-point Likert scale ranging from 1 (*Strongly Disagree*) to 5 (*Strongly Agree*) that measures perceived benefits of barebacking. The BOBS has been shown to have strong psychometric properties with an alpha coefficient of .90. Construct validity has been established using exploratory factor analytic methods, which demonstrated that 9 of the 14 items loaded on one factor for this scale (Halkitis, Parsons and Wilton, 2003b). In the present investigation, an internal consistency reliability of .92 was found. Sample items included: "Barebacking increases intimacy between men," "Barebacking makes sex more romantic," "Barebacking is sexier than sex with condoms," and "Barebacking affirms love between men."

Qualitative Measures

For the larger-scale longitudinal study, a subset of approximately 100 qualitative interviews was randomly selected for transcription based on each of the five frequently used club drugs. In the present investigation, 24 qualitative interviews (12 from the Black participants and 12 from the Latino participants) from the larger set were randomly selected for qualitative data analysis.

The Baseline Qualitative Protocol guided the discussion for the qualitative component of the study; probes were used for each question to obtain in-depth data regarding the constructs that were assessed. Some of the protocol's questions included: (1) Tell me about the first time you tried (Frequently Used Drug or FUD); (2) Tell me about your use of (FUD); (3) How has your use of (FUD) changed over time?; (4) What do you like about using (FUD) or what do you get out of using this drug?; (5) How does (FUD) affect your sex behaviors or what you do sexually?; (6) How do certain combinations of club drugs and other drugs affect your sex behaviors or what you do sexually?; and (7) What are your thoughts about barebacking? What does it mean to you? For the purposes of the qualitative interview, barebacking was defined for the participants as "unprotected anal intercourse that you've had intentionally, not, for example, because the condom broke or you were high and then regretted it."

RESULTS

Quantitative Findings

A total of 450 men completed baseline measures for the study. Of this number, 14.7% ($n = 66$) identified as Black, 19.8% ($n = 89$) as Latino, 5.3% ($n = 24$) as Asian/Pacific Islander, 51.1% ($n = 230$) as White,

6.2% (*n* = 28) as Mixed Heritage/Race, 0.4% (*n* = 2) as Native American, and 2.4% (*n* = 11) as Other. The purpose of the quantitative analyses was to consider the differences between Black and Latino men in relation to the remainder of the sample. Thus, we trichotomized the data into three racial/ethnic groups: Black (*n* = 66), Latino (*n* = 89), and Other (*n* = 295).

Sociodemographic Characteristics

Table 1 provides the sociodemographic characteristics of the sample. In terms of Black men, the mean age of the participants was 33.55 (SD = 7.44, range = 18-48). The majority of the Black men identified as gay (84.8%, *n* = 56) followed by bisexual (15.2%, *n* = 10). In regard to gender, one Black male participant identified as transgender (1.5%, *n* = 1), with the remainder of the participants identifying as male (98.5%, *n* = 65). In terms of self-reported HIV status, 50.0% (*n* = 33) of the Black men identified as HIV-positive, 40.9% (*n* = 27) as HIV-negative, and 9.1% (*n* = 6) were unaware of their HIV status. About one-third of the Black men completed high school/GED (28.8%, *n* = 19), while less than half reported some college/Associate's degree (40.9%, *n* = 27) or a Bachelor's degree (19.7%, *n* = 13). Fifty-two percent (*n* = 34) of the Black men were employed full- or part-time. The primary three income levels for the Black men were: (1) Less than $10,000 (33.3%, *n* = 22), (2) $10,000 to $19,999 (21.2%, *n* = 14), and (3) $20,000 to $29,999 (19.7%, *n* = 13).

For the Latino men, the mean age was 30.64 (SD = 7.04, range = 18-47). Approximately 80% (*n* = 72) identified as gay and 20% (*n* = 17) as bisexual. One hundred percent (*n* = 89) of the Latino men identified as male in relation to gender. In terms of self-reported HIV status, 34.8% (*n* = 31) of the Latino men identified as HIV-positive, 61.8% (*n* = 55) as HIV-negative, and 3.4% (*n* = 3) were unaware of their HIV status. Slightly less than half of the Latino men completed some college/Associate's degree (47.2%, *n* = 42), while 18% (*n* = 16) acquired a high school diploma/GED or Bachelor's degree (19.1%, *n* = 17). About 54% (*n* = 48) of the Latino men were employed full- or part-time. The primary three income levels of the Latino men were: (1) $20,000 to $29,999 (27.0%, *n* = 24), (2) Less than $10,000 (22.5%, *n* = 20), and (3) $10,000 to $19,999 (18.0%, *n* = 16).

For the remainder of the sample, categorized as Other men, the mean age was 33.28 (SD = 8.20, range = 18-67). The majority of the men identified as gay (90.8%, *n* = 268) with fewer as bisexual (9.2%, *n* = 27).

TABLE 1. Participant Demographic Characteristics

Variable	Black % (Number)	Latino % (Number)	Other % (Number)
Sexual Identity			
Gay	84.8%(56)	80.9% (72)	90.8% (268)
Bisexual	15.2% (10)	19.1% (17)	9.2% (27)
Gender			
Male	98.5% (65)	100% (89)	100% (295)
Transgender	1.5% (1)	0% (0)	0% (0)
Current HIV Status			
HIV-Negative	40.9% (27)	61.8% (55)	65.1% (192)
HIV-Positive	50.0% (33)	34.8% (31)	29.2% (86)
Don't Know	9.1% (6)	3.4% (3)	5.8% (17)
Educational Background			
Did Not Complete HS	3.0% (2)	5.6% (5)	1.4% (4)
High School Diploma/GED	28.8% (19)	18.0% (15)	6.1% (18)
Some College/Assoc. Degree	40.9% (27)	47.2% (42)	29.2% (86)
Bachelor's Degree	19.7% (13)	19.1% (17)	45.8% (135)
Graduate Degree	7.6% (5)	10.1% (9)	17.6% (52)
Current Employment Status			
Full-Time	28.8% (19)	28.1% (25)	42.7% (126)
Part-Time	22.7% (15)	25.8% (23)	22.4% (66)
Disability (not working)	10.6% (7)	9.0% (8)	6.1% (18)
Disability (working off books)	4.5% (3)	4.5% (4)	3.7% (11)
Unemployed (Student)	7.6% (5)	16.9% (15)	3.7% (11)
Unemployed (Other)	25.8% (17)	15.7% (14)	21.0% (62)
Total Personal Income			
Less than $10,000	33.3% (22)	22.5% (20)	11.9% (35)
$10,000 to $19,999	21.2% (14)	18.0% (16)	13.9% (41)
$20,000 to $29,999	19.7% (13)	27.0% (24)	11.9% (35)
$30,000 to $39,999	10.6% (7)	9.0% (8)	17.3% (51)
$40,000 to $49,999	7.6% (5)	10.1% (9)	11.2% (33)
$50,000 to $74,999	6.1% (4)	5.6% (5)	21.4% (63)
$75,000 to $99,999	1.5% (1)	3.4% (3)	4.4% (13)
$100,000 or more	0% (0)	2.2% (2)	6.8% (20)

In terms of gender, one hundred percent ($n = 295$) identified as male. More than half of the men reported being HIV-negative (65.1, $n = 192$), followed by HIV-positive (29.2%, $n = 86$), with the remainder of the men unaware of their HIV status (5.8%, $n = 17$). Most of the men completed a Bachelor's degree (45.8%, $n = 135$), some college/Associate's degree (29.2%, $n = 86$) or graduate degree (17.6%, $n = 52$). The majority of the men were employed either full- or part-time (65.1%, $n = 192$). The main three income levels of the men were: (1) $50,000 to $74,000 (21.4%, $n = 63$), (2) $30,000 to $39,999 (17.3%, $n = 51$), and (3) $10,000 to $19,999 (13.9%, $n = 41$).

There were significant racial/ethnic differences in the sample in relation to sociodemographic characteristics. Sexual identity differed by race/ethnicity in that significantly more Black and Latino men, as compared to Other men, identified as bisexual ($\chi^2 (2) = 7.14$, $p = .02$). Specifically, 15.2% of the Black men and 19.1% of the Latino men identified as bisexual as compared to 9.2% of the Other men. However, in terms of behaviors, while 60% of the Black bisexual men and 56% of the Other bisexual men reported sex with women in the last four months, only 47% of the Latino bisexual men reported this behavior.

In relation to age, both Black men and Other men were slightly older than Latino men ($F(2, 447) = 4.19$, $p = .02$). In particular, Latino men were 31-years-old (SD = 7.04), Black men were 34-years-old (SD = 7.44), and Other men were 33-years-old (SD = 8.20). In terms of HIV status, significantly more Black and Latino men reported being HIV-positive as compared to Other men ($\chi^2 (4) = 14.45$, $p < .01$). Specifically, while 50.0% of the Black men and 34.8% of the Latino men self-reported being HIV-positive, only 29.2% of the Other men reported an HIV-positive status. Further, significantly more Black men as compared to the Latino men and Other men were unaware of their HIV status. In particular, 9.1% of the Black men, 3.4% of the Latino men, and 5.8% of the Other men were unaware of their HIV status.

With regard to educational background, there were significant differences between Black and Latino men in comparison to Other men ($\chi^2 (8) = 64.39$, $p < .001$). Specifically, while 45.8% of Other men obtained a minimum of a bachelor's level education, only 19.7% of Black men and 19.1% of Latino men reported a bachelor's degree as their highest educational level. Similarly, in terms of total personal income during the last year, significant racial/ethnic differences were found in the sample ($\chi^2 (14) = 56.85$, $p < .001$). Specifically, 74% of Black men reported an income of less than $30,000 per year, 69% of Latino men reported incomes in this range, while only 38% of all others reported this level of income.

Characteristics of Club Drug Use

For the purposes of the analyses, the sample was categorized as non-users, binge users, and chronic users of the club drug substances. Racial/ethnic differences in club drug use were found in the sample. For example, significantly more Latino and Other men reported binge use of crystal methamphetamine as compared to Black men (χ^2 (4) = 11.58, p = .02). Specifically, while 59.6% of Latino men and 63.1% of Other men reported binge use of crystal methamphetamine, only 43.9% of Black men reported binge use of this substance. Similarly, differential rates of MDMA or ecstasy use by race/ethnicity were noted in the sample (χ^2 (4) = 22.83, p < .001). Specifically, while 69.7% of Latino men and 75.5% of Other men reported binge use of ecstasy, only 46.2% of Black men reported binge use of this substance.

With regard to cocaine, the likelihood of chronic use was greater in Black and Latino men as compared to Other men; however, all three groups demonstrated about the same rate of binge use of this substance (χ^2 (4) = 18.81, p < .001). Specifically, while 22.7% of Black men and 20.2% of Latino men reported chronic use of cocaine, only 8.5% of Other men reported chronic use of this substance. Further, 66.7% of Black men, 61.8% of Latino men, and 67.1% of Other men reported binge use of cocaine. In contrast, significantly more Latino and Other men demonstrated higher rates of binge use of ketamine than Black men (χ^2 (4) = 25.82, p < .001). For example, while only 24.2% of Black men reported binge use of ketamine, 56.2% of Latino men and 58.0% of Other men reported binge use of this substance. No significant racial/ethnic differences were found in the use of GHB.

Characteristics of Barebacking

For the entire sample, we sought to assess whether rates of barebacking with men of differing HIV serostatus varied. Results demonstrated that rates were consistent across the three types of serostatus partners (i.e., the men in our sample reported equivalent rates of barebacking with HIV-positive, HIV-negative, and HIV status unknown partners). The overall reported means were as follows: Mean frequency of barebacking with HIV-positive partners (M = 1.97, SD =

12.28), HIV-negative (M = 2.84, SD = 16.32), and HIV status unknown (M = 3.35, SD = 15.06).

Next, we sought to determine whether race and HIV status was related to the frequency with which men engaged in barebacking. Table 2 provides the mean number of reported bareback sexual encounters as a function of participant's serostatus and in relation to partner's serostatus. A 3 (participant's serostatus: HIV-positive, HIV-negative, and HIV status unknown) × 3 (partner's serostatus: HIV-positive, HIV-negative, and HIV status unknown) analysis of variance demonstrated a significant effect for HIV status of participant (F(2, 441) = 5.08, p < .01); however, no effect for race, or the interaction of race by HIV status of the individual, was found. Specifically, HIV-positive men reported significantly more frequent barebacking with HIV-positive partners as compared to HIV-negative men with these partners (p < .001). Further, there was a trend towards significance with HIV-positive men reporting more bareback sex with HIV-positive partners than HIV status unknown men reported with HIV-positive partners (p = .06). However, when we examined the frequencies of barebacking with HIV-negative and HIV status unknown partners, there was no effect for race, HIV status of participant, or the interaction of the two.

Finally, in terms of the Benefits of Barebacking Scale, there was an interactive effect for race and HIV status (F(4, 421) = 2.43, p = .05). The analyses indicated that Latino men of HIV unknown status perceived greater benefits of barebacking as compared to any other group according to HIV status or race/ethnicity.

Qualitative Findings

Thematic coding was used to analyze the data from the qualitative interviews based on procedures outlined by Miles and Huberman (1994). One of the major tenets of this approach "affirms[s] the existence and importance of the subjective, the phenomenological, the meaning-making at the center of social life" (p. 4). As such, the objective here was focused on "capturing the 'essence'" of the narratives to identify themes and factors associated with perceptions and phenomenological meanings attached to barebacking, club drug use, and the intersection of the two sets of behaviors. In the proceeding section, qualitative data will be described according to the participant's race/ethnicity, gender, HIV status, and frequently used club drug.

TABLE 2. Barebacking Behavior Across Partner Type and Race

Participant Serostatus	Partner Serostatus		
HIV-Positive Men			
	Positive	Negative	Unknown
Black	0.64	0.00	0.00
	(SD = 2.03)	(SD = 0.00)	(SD = 0.00)
Latino	8.03	0.53	0.00
	(SD = 38.64)	(SD = 2.81)	(SD = 0.00)
Other	5.98	0.33	0.53
	(SD = 14.56)	(SD = 2.24)	(SD = 1.59)
HIV-Negative Men			
	Positive	Negative	Unknown
Black	0.18	2.41	0.17
	(SD = 0.77)	(SD = 5.99)	(SD = 0.41)
Latino	1.06	2.40	0.67
	(SD = 4.30)	(SD = 6.85)	(SD = 1.15)
Other	8.12	1.40	4.18
	(SD = 35.45)	(SD = 4.78)	(SD = 8.61)
HIV Status Unknown Men			
	Positive	Negative	Unknown
Black	1.00	1.63	0.00
	(SD = 3.51)	(SD = 5.15)	(SD = 0.00)
Latino	8.71	6.64	1.67
	(SD = 37.92)	(SD = 22.63)	(SD = 2.89)
Other	5.49	1.17	5.65
	(SD = 13.54)	(SD = 4.76)	(SD = 20.49)

PERCEPTIONS OF BAREBACKING

One consistent aspect of the sexual narratives of the Black and Latino gay and bisexual men related to the familiarity with the term "barebacking." Most of the men ascribed differential usage and meaning to the term, including most commonly defining barebacking as "anal intercourse without a condom," "Having sex without a condom," or "Fucking without a condom." According to one participant, "Yeah, I just always called it raw dog. I didn't know barebacking. Different people have different slang." This participant further discussed his decision-making process regarding the selection of a bareback sex partner, "Hmmm, like, you can look for something as subtle as the look in their face (Latino male, age 31, HIV status unknown, Ecstasy).

Many of the Black and Latino men in the qualitative narratives discussed their perceptions of the barebacking phenomena, particularly as related to complex interrelationships involving norms, attitudes, and behaviors:

> Total trust. A situation where you totally trust; like a marriage situation. Before I found out I was HIV-positive, I didn't know what a condom was. Now, I know my HIV status and I would never want to put that on anybody else emotionally or mentally. So, I make sure that the chances are nil for them to ever contract it. (Black male, age 42, HIV-positive, Cocaine)

Some of the participants affirmed strong values about the importance of safer sex norms. For example, one commercial sex worker contended, "They [clients] always–a lot of them ask me [to have bareback sex] and I'm like 'No. If you don't want to use a condom, then go find somebody else.'" (Latino male, age 18, HIV-negative, Cocaine). Another participant commented:

> I haven't and you shouldn't do that [engage in bareback sex] unless you know that both of you aren't HIV [positive] . . . If you both are positive, you shouldn't do it because you are going to get re-infected. (Black male, age 37, HIV-positive, Cocaine)

In contrast, some men of color discussed their experiences of engaging in the practice of barebacking. One participant commented, "I bareback every once in a while with a casual partner" (Black male, age 40, HIV positive, Cocaine). According to another participant, "Well, it's okay, as long as they [casual partners] don't cum inside me" (Latino male, age 29, HIV-negative, Cocaine). Further, one of the men, in response to an interviewer's comment, "Even if a condom was like right here . . ." responded: "No, I wouldn't [use a condom] 'cause condoms are like near my bed in a fish bowl. I don't even think about the condoms" (Black male, age 24, HIV status unknown, Cocaine).

MEANINGS OF SEX AND CLUB DRUG USE

Many of the Black and Latino men in their sexual narratives discussed the subjective meaning of condomless sex in their lives. Thus, the act of sex between two men was experienced as a form of intimacy and emotional connectedness to a sexual partner. Significantly, some men of color discussed the desire and centrality of bareback sex, not as a deficit, as an affirmation of gay male sexuality. According to one participant:

> Because I love my partner and we both decided that [bareback sex] is what we want to do. So, it was a mutual agreement. Yeah, there's a difference, because I do care about him. I want to be up in him. I don't want a condom on. I want to feel everything. (Black male, age 31, HIV-positive, Cocaine)

The negotiation of dual identities, racial and gay, as gay men of color often has been connected to larger cultural norms involving racism in gay communities and homophobia in Black communities (Greene, 1997). As a result, Black and Latino men have experienced multiple forms of disconnection, which has, at times, influenced their sexual behavior (Diaz, 1997). One of the men, for example, elaborated on the difficulty of having a gay identity:

> Maybe it's just dealing with 'cause, even though I want to be bisexual . . . maybe feel more comfortable around a lot of gay men at one time. Feeling less guilty about what I'm doing. (Black male, age 34, HIV status unknown, Cocaine)

Further, the complexities of the negotiation of condom use through non-verbal cues was intricately related to sex: "Well, because I kind of pulled [condoms] out, so right when I reached for them, we didn't have to speak any words about it" (Black male, age 36, HIV-positive, Ketamine).

Yet, some men of color discussed how the act of sex served as an affirmation of their physical attractiveness and sexual desirability. One participant described a sexual experience with a 36-year-old, Black casual partner:

> The fact that he [casual partner] was all over me. He was very attractive. He's got all of the right things: he's responsible, he's hard-working, he has a new car. I felt really good about myself. (Black male, age 42, HIV-positive, Cocaine)

While, at the same time, for some Black and Latino men, sexual desirability often was connected to their perceptions and decision-making processes regarding a casual partner's HIV status. In the words of one participant, "I would predict that he is already HIV positive and very careful, or he is HIV negative and very careful" (Black male, age 22, HIV-negative, Crystal Methamphetamine). For other men, the meaning attached to the act of sex was discussed in relation to the negotiation of HIV disclosure with sexual partners: "No he doesn't know [my HIV status], but we don't do anything so he doesn't need to know" (Black male, age 37, HIV-positive, Cocaine).

Based on the sexual narratives, many of the Black and Latino men discussed how club drug use was connected to the act and subjective meaning of sex with their sexual partners. One participant remarked, "It makes me a little bit more daring to do things that I wouldn't really do normally" (Black male, age 35, HIV-positive, Cocaine). Another individual discussed how the use of club drugs had an impact on their sexual roles assumed during sex: "Um, I think I'm more topping when I'm high" (Black, age 35, HIV-negative, Cocaine). Further, one participant described sex while using cocaine with a 34-year-old, Black HIV status unknown casual partner:

> We were watching videos, doing a few lines [of cocaine] and then clothes started coming off. From touching to kissing, then from kissing to oral sex to anal sex. We used condoms for anal sex but not for oral sex. (Black, age 42, HIV-positive, Cocaine)

While some gay men of color discussed the practice of engaging in unprotected sexual behaviors, including bareback sex, while using club drugs, others expressed how the use of these substances often served as a facilitator to have sex:

> Sometimes when I smoke [cocaine] . . . I can take my first hit of it and I just start to drop my pants for somebody and he could start sucking my cock. (Black male, age 28, HIV status unknown, Cocaine)

> I had put some coke on the head of my dick and had him [partner] lick it off, and that kind of turned me on even more. (Latino male, age 35, HIV-positive, Cocaine)

> It helps me get into the mood. It relaxes me, especially when you are having sex and you've been with your partner for a long time. When I haven't had sex with him in a while, I'm nervous when we do it. I'm thinking, 'Can I get hard?' 'Is it going to be good?' 'Am I going to like it?'" (Black male, age 31, HIV-positive, Cocaine)

A number of the Black and Latino men discussed how polydrug use, or the combination of club drugs, other illicit drugs, and alcohol, had an impact on their sexual behavior:

> Ecstasy is wonderful because it smoothes out that hardness from the coke and it's a very flowing type of liquid feel. And, I've noticed that I get the feeling that I'm making love. And, I hold the person even more and I notice that they are holding me more. (Latino male, age 22, HIV-negative)

One participant described their experience at a sex party while using ketamine:

> Oh, it was like a group of people, it was a sex party and everybody was doing different things and everybody was trying different things, so I was just trying it. (Latino male, age 38, HIV status unknown, Cocaine)

Another participant described using cocaine while having bareback sex with a 27-year-old, Latino male who was an anonymous sex partner:

> It was like understood when we got to my place it [bareback sex] was going to happen so, we got undressed when we got there, and

we did some more lines. It's very risky behavior, I mean I don't know the person. I don't know their HIV status, and I'm having unprotected sex. (Black male, age 43, HIV status unknown, Cocaine)

DISCUSSION

The purpose of this exploratory investigation was to examine barebacking, club drug use, and meanings of sex in a community-based sample of Black and Latino gay and bisexual (BLGB) men. Our first major finding demonstrated that there were significant racial and ethnic differences in relation to the sociodemographic characteristics in the sample. Specifically, while Black and Latino men, as compared to the remainder of the sample, were more likely to report an HIV-positive serostatus, Black men were significantly more likely to be unaware of their HIV status. Consistent with current epidemiological data (CDC, 2003) and other empirical studies (Koblin et al., 2000; Valleroy et al., 2000), this finding suggests that the increasing prevalence and disproportionate rate of HIV among BLGB men further substantiates the link between the emergence of club drug use with an increased risk for HIV seroconversion in this group of men. Significantly, in a recent investigation (Carragher et al., 2004) with this sample, 43.8% of Black gay and bisexual men self-reporting an HIV-negative status at the baseline assessment seroconverted during the course of the study.

Second, Black and Latino men demonstrated more likelihood to identify as bisexual than the overall sample. Similarly, this finding is consistent with recent research (Mays, Cochran and Zamudio, 2004; Munoz-Laboy, 2004) and underscores the importance of developing specific HIV prevention strategies for Black and Latino bisexual men that focus on the adoption and maintenance of safer sex behaviors. For example, prevention strategies need to account for how Black and Latino bisexual men may be a more invisible group and disconnected from traditional prevention programs that focus on gay men. Further, BLGB men are at risk for experiencing stigma and race- and gay-related stress, due to racism and homophobia (Crawford et al., 2004; Diaz et al., 2001).

In terms of bisexuality and sexual intercourse with women, the present investigation showed that 60% of Black bisexual men, 56% of Other bisexual men, and 47% of Latino bisexual men reported sex with women in the past four months prior to assessment. In contrast, Bimbi and Parsons (2005) found no significant relationship between bisexuality and sexual intercourse with women, although this finding corroborates with the work of Montgomery et al. (2003). While current epidemiological data demonstrates that heterosexual transmission of HIV has increased (CDC, 2004b), especially for women of color, empirical evidence indicates that a multitude of risk factors relate to these disproportionate rates for Black women including but not limited to cultural factors (i.e., condom use beliefs), behavioral factors (i.e., heterosexual contact, bisexuality, injection drug use), structural factors (i.e., poverty, health disparities), and social factors (i.e., race- and gender-related stress) (McNair and Prather, 2004). Nonetheless, with the insurgence of the "Down Low" phenomenon, Black men's same-gender identities and behavior have been pejoratively constructed and ascribed as the predominant vector of HIV transmission for Black women.

In accordance with recent investigations (Halkitis, Parsons and Wilton, 2003a), empirical evidence from this study suggests an increasing prevalence of club drug use in men of color from the New York Metropolitan area. Yet, previous research indicated that club drugs were primarily used in White communities from the Western region of the U.S. (Rawson, Gonzalez and Brethen, 2002). Specifically, in the present study, Black and Latino men, as compared to the overall sample, demonstrated more chronic use of cocaine, while Latino and Other men reported higher rates of binge use of crystal methamphetamine, ecstasy, and ketamine than Black men. Further, the qualitative data showed that many of the Black and Latino men engaged in polydrug use, which often influenced their sexual behavior. Although Halkitis et al. (2005) found that barebackers, as compared to non-barebackers, reported GHB use, our findings showed no significant differences in GHB use across racial/ethnic groups. This disparity may be due to the small number of GHB users in this sample.

Comparable to current HIV prevention studies of the sexual behavior of MSM (Mansergh et al., 2002), we found that HIV-positive men, regardless of race/ethnicity, engaged in bareback sex more than HIV-negative men, particularly with other HIV-positive sexual partners (Halkitis et al., 2004). This finding is significant because it indicates similar patterns of bareback sexual behavior across racial/ethnic groups in MSM. However, the qualitative findings from this study suggest that the act of bareback sex holds differential cultural and phenomenological meanings for Black and Latino men. Thus, current HIV prevention strategies must move beyond traditional social cognitive theoretical paradigms and incorporate the language (Mays et al., 1992) and racial/cultural conceptual worldviews of men of color.

Further, we found that Latino men who were unaware of their HIV status perceived greater benefits of barebacking than any other group according to race/ethnicity and HIV status. One plausible reason for this finding relates to the social construction of masculinity in Latino/a culture, particularly with respect to the socialization processes of Latino men. For example, Diaz (1998) contends that the internalization of a "machismo discourse" for Latino men connects masculinity with sexual risk behavior. Thus, the act of bareback sex for Latino men holds specific cultural and phenomenological meanings and, according to Diaz, relates to four psychological processes–pleasure, connection, affirmation, and exchange–that have an impact on their sexual behavior. Yet, a dearth of HIV prevention research and interventions has incorporated cultural conceptions of sexual behavior for Latino men.

LIMITATIONS

The findings of this exploratory investigation should be viewed in relation to the correlational nature of the data, thus causal implications should not be inferred. Further, one major limitation of the present study relates to the period of recall and self-report nature of the data and potential socially desirable responses of sexual and drug risk behavior, especially with respect to under- or over-reporting of risk behavior. However, ACASI has been shown to increase the proportion of individuals reporting sexual behaviors and illicit drug use, as well as provide greater respondent privacy and remove barriers to honest responding, such as embarrassment, feedback from facial expressions of the interviewer, and other social influences (Macalino et al., 2002).

Future investigations should examine inter- and intra-group differences in relation to cultural worldviews for Black and Latino men in relation to the constructs assessed. For example, African, Caribbean (English-, Spanish-, and French-speaking), as well as Central and South American MSM often have been neglected in HIV prevention research. Specifically, with the increasing shift in demographic trends of Black and Latino individuals immigrating to the U.S., research needs to explore the sociocultural factors that may have an impact on the interaction between drug use and HIV sexual risk behavior including immigration experiences, acculturation, language, gender role socialization, and social support (Harris-Hastick, 2001).

REFERENCES

Bimbi, D. & Parsons, J.T. (2005), Barebacking among Internet based male sex workers. *J. Gay & Lesbian Psychotherapy*, 9(3/4):85-106.

Bochow, M. (1998), The importance of contextualizing research: An analysis of data from the German gay press survey. *J. Psychology & Human Sexuality*, 10:37-58.

Carballo-Dieguez, A. & Dolezal, C. (1996), HIV risk behaviors and obstacles to condom use among Puerto Rican men in New York City who have sex with men. *American J. Public Health*, 86:1619-1622.

Carragher, D., Halkitis, P.N., Mourgues, P. & Burke, A., (2004), *Seroconversion and Club Drug Use: A Contextual Understanding*. Paper presented at the annual meeting of the American Psychological Association, Honolulu, HI, August 1.

Centers for Disease Control and Prevention (2001), HIV incidence among young men who have sex with men–Seven U.S. cities, 1994-2000. *Morbidity & Mortality Weekly Report*, 50:440-444.

Centers for Disease Control and Prevention (2002), Unrecognized HIV infection, risk behaviors, and perceptions of risk among young Black men who have sex with men–Six U.S. cities, 1994-1998. *Morbidity & Mortality Weekly Report*, 51:733-736.

Centers for Disease Control and Prevention (2003), HIV/STD risks in young men who have sex with men who do not disclose their sexual orientation–Six U.S. cities, 1994-2000. *Morbidity & Mortality Weekly Report*, 52:81-85.

Centers for Disease Control and Prevention (2004a), Cases of HIV infection and AIDS in the United States, by race and ethnicity, 1998-2002. *HIV/AIDS Surveillance Supplemental Report*, 10:1-38.

Centers for Disease Control and Prevention (2004b), Heterosexual transmission of HIV–29 states, 1999-2002. *Morbidity & Mortality Weekly Report*, 53:125-129.

Chen, S.Y., Gibson, S., Katz, M.H., Klausner, J.D., Dilley, J.W., Schwarcz, S.K. et al. (2002), Continuing increases in sexual risk behavior and sexually transmitted diseases among men who have sex with men: San Francisco, California, 1999-2001. *American J. Public Health*, 92:1387-1388.

Chesney, M.A., Barrett, D.C. & Stall, R. (1998), Histories of substance use and risk behavior: Precursors to HIV seroconversion in homosexual men. *American J. Public Health*, 88:113-116.

Clatts, M. (2004), *A Drug and Sex Risk Profile of Four MSM Groups in New York City: Have Existing Public Health Interventions Failed!?* Paper presented at the National Institute of Drug Abuse/CAMCODA Conference, March 1-2.

Colfax, G., Vittinghoff, E., Husnik, M., Huang, E., Buchbinder, S., Chesney, M. et al. (2004), *Substance Use During Sex Is Associated with High-Risk Behavior: An Episode-Specific Analysis Among the EXPLORE Study Cohort*. Paper presented at the National Institute of Drug Abuse/CAMCODA Conference, March 1-2.

Crawford, I., Allison, K., Zamboni, B.D. & Soto, T. (2002), The influence of dual-identity development on the psychosocial functioning of African-American gay and bisexual men. *J. Sex Research*, 39:179-189.

Creswell, J. (2002), *Research Design: Qualitative, Quantitative, and Mixed Methods Approaches, 2nd Edition*. Thousand Oaks, CA: Sage Publications.

Deren, S., Beardsley, M., Coyle, S. & Singer, M. (1998), HIV serostatus and risk behaviors in a multisite sample of drug users. *J. Psychoactive Drugs*, 30:239-245.

Diaz, R.M. (1998), *Latino Gay Men and HIV: Culture, Sexuality, and Risk Behavior.* New York: Routledge.

Diaz, R.M., Ayala, G., Bein, E., Henne, J. & Marin, B.V. (2001), The impact of homophobia, poverty, and racism on the mental health of gay and bisexual Latino men: Findings from three US cities. *American J. Public Health*, 91:927-932.

Diaz, R.M., Heckert, A.L. and Sanchez, J. (2004), *Fabulous Effects/Disastrous Consequences.* Paper presented at the National Institute of Drug Abuse/CAMCODA Conference, March 1-2.

Dolezal, C., Meyer-Bahlburg, H.F.L., Remien, R.H. & Petkova, E. (1997), Substance use during sex and sensation seeking as predictors of sexual risk behavior among HIV+ and HIV− gay men. *AIDS & Behavior*, 1:19-28.

Fuller, C.M., Absalon, J., Ompad, D.C., Blaney, S., Galea, S. & Vlahov, D. (2004), *Correlates of Injection Drug Use Among Illicit Drug-Using MSM: Implications for Future Research and Intervention Strategies.* Paper presented at the National Institute of Drug Abuse/CAMCODA Conference, March 1-2.

Greene, B. (1997), Ethnic minority lesbians and gay men: Mental health and treatment issues. In: *Ethnic and Cultural Diversity Among Lesbians and Gay Men*, ed. B. Greene. Thousand Oaks, CA: Sage Publications, pp. 216-239.

Greenwood, G.L., White, E.W., Page-Shafer, K., Bein, E., Osmond, D.H., Paul, J. et al. (2001), Correlates of heavy substance use among young gay and bisexual men: The San Francisco Young Men's Health Study. *Drug & Alcohol Dependence*, 61: 105-112.

Halkitis, P.N., Parsons, J.T. & Wilton, L. (2003a), An exploratory study of contextual and situational factors related to methamphetamine use among gay and bisexual men in New York City. *J. Drug Issues*, 33:413-432.

Halkitis, P.N., Parsons, J.T. & Wilton, L. (2003b), Barebacking among gay and bisexual men in New York City: Explanations for the emergency of intentional unsafe behavior. *Archives Sexual Behavior*, 32:351-357.

Halkitis, P.N., Wilton, L., & Parsons, J.T. & Hoff, C. (2004), Correlates of sexual risk-taking behavior among HIV seropositive gay men in seroconcordant primary partner relationships. *Psychology, Health, & Medicine*, 9:99-113.

Halkitis, P.N., Wilton, L., Wolitski, R.J., Parsons, J.T., Hoff, C. & Bimbi, D. (2005), Barebacking identity among HIV-positive gay and bisexual men: Demographic, psychological, and behavior correlates. *AIDS*(Supp1): 527-535.

Harris-Hastick, E.F. (2001), Substance abuse issues among English-speaking Caribbean people of African ancestry. In: *Ethnocultural Factors in Substance Abuse Treatment*, ed. S.L.A. Straussner. New York: Guilford Press, pp. 52-74.

Klein, M. & Kramer, F. (2004), Rave drugs: Pharmacological considerations. *AANA Journal*, 72:61-67.

Knox, S., Kippax, S., Crawford, J., Prestage, G. & Van de Ven, P. (1999), Non-prescription drug use by gay men in Sydney, Melbourne and Brisbane. *Drug & Alcohol Review*, 18:425-433.

Koblin, B.A., Torian, L.V., Gulin, V., Ren, L., MacKellar, D.A. & Valleroy, L.A. (2000), High prevalence of HIV infection among young men who have sex with men in New York City. *AIDS*, 14:1793-1800.

Mansergh, G., Marks, G., Colfax, G., Guzman, R., Rader, M. & Buchbinder, S. (2002), Barebacking in a diverse sample of men who have sex with men. *AIDS*, 16:653-659.

Macalino, G.E., Celentano, D.D., Latkin, C., Strathdee, S.A. & Vlahov, D. (2002), Risk behaviors by audio computer-assisted self-interviews among HIV-seropositive and HIV-seronegative injection drug users. *AIDS Education & Prevention*, 14:367-378.

Mays, V.M., Cochran, S.D., Bellinger, G. & Smith, R.G. (1992), The language of Black gay men's sexual behavior: Implications for AIDS risk reduction. *J. Sex Research*, 29:425-434.

Mays, V.M., Cochran, S.D. & Zamudio, A. (2004), HIV prevention research: Are we meeting the needs of African American men who have sex with men? *J. Black Psychology*, 30:78-105.

McDowell, D. (2000), Gay men, lesbians and substances of abuse and the "club and circuit party scene": What clinicians should know. *J. Gay & Lesbian Psychotherapy*, 3(3/4):37-57. Reprinted in: *Addictions in the Gay and Lesbian Community*, eds. J.R. Guss & J. Drescher. New York: The Haworth Press, 2000, pp. 37-57.

McKirnan, D.J., Ostrow, D.G. & Hope, B. (1996), Sex, drugs, and escape: A psychological model of HIV-risk sexual behaviors. *AIDS Care*, 8:655-669.

McNair, L.D. & Prather, C.M. (2004), African women and AIDS: Factors influencing risk and reaction to HIV disease. *J. Black Psychology*, 30:106-123.

Metsch, L.R., McCoy, C.B., Lai, S. & Miles, C. (1998), Continuing risk behaviors among HIV-seropositive chronic drug users in Miami, Florida. *AIDS & Behavior*, 2:161-169.

Miles, M.B. & Huberman, M. (1994). *Qualitative Data Analysis: An Expanded Sourcebook, 2nd Edition*. Thousand Oaks, CA: Sage Publications.

Montgomery, J.P., Mokotoff, E.D., Gentry, A.C. & Blair, J.M. (2003), The extent of bisexual behavior in HIV-infected men and implications for transmission to their female sex partners. *AIDS Care*, 15:829-837.

Munoz-Laboy, M.A. (2004), Beyond "MSM": Sexual desire among bisexually-active Latino men in New York City. *Sexualities*, 7:55-80.

Parsons, J.T. & Halkitis, P.N. (2002), Sexual and drug using practices of HIV+ men who frequent commercial and public sex environments. *AIDS Care*, 14:815-826.

Peterson, J.L. & Carballo-Dieguez, A. (2000), HIV prevention among African-American and Latino men who have sex with men. In: *Handbook of HIV Prevention*, eds. J.L. Peterson & R.J. Carballo-Dieguez. Secaucus, NJ: Kluwer Academic Publishers, pp. 217-224.

Rawson, R.A., Gonzales, R. & Brethen, P. (2002), Treatment of methamphetamine use disorders: An update. *J. Substance Abuse Treatment*, 23:145-150.

Romanelli, F. & Smith, K.M. (2004), Recreational use of sildenafil by HIV-positive and HIV-negative homosexual/bisexual males. *Annals Pharmacotherapy*, 38: 1024-1030.

Ross, R.W., Wodak, A., Gold, J. & Miller, M.E. (1992), Differences across sexual orientation on HIV risk behaviours in injecting drug users. *AIDS Care*, 4:139-148.

Stall, R., Paul, J.P., Greenwood, G., Pollack, L.M., Bein, E., Crosby, G.M. et al. (2001), Alcohol use, drug use and alcohol-related problems among men who have sex with men: The Urban Men's Health Study. *Addiction*, 96:1589-1601.

Stall, R. & Purcell, D.W. (2000), Intertwining epidemics: A review of research on substance use among men who have sex with men and its connection to the AIDS epidemic. *AIDS & Behavior*, 4:181-192.

Valleroy, L.A., MacKellar, D.A., Karon, J.M., Rosen, D.H., McFarland, W., Shehan, D.A. et al. (2000), HIV prevalence and associated risks in young men who have sex with men. *J. American Medical Association*, 284:198-204.

Vargo, S., Agronick, G., O'Donnell, L. & Stueve, A. (2004), Using peer recruitment and Orasure to increase HIV testing. *American J. Public Health*, 94:29-31.

Watters, J.K. & Biernacki, P. (1989), Targeted sampling: Options for the study of hidden populations. *Social Problems*, 36:416-430.

Wilton, L. (2001), Perceived health risks and psychosocial factors as predictors of sexual risk-taking within HIV-positive gay male seroconcordant couples. *Dissertation Abstracts International*, 61(7-B):3867.

Wolitski, R.J., Valdisserri, R.O., Denning, P.H. & Levine, W.C. (2001), Are we headed for a resurgence in the HIV epidemic among men who have sex with men? *American J. Public Health*, 91:883-888.

Wright, E.M. (2001), Substance abuse in African American communities. In: *Ethnocultural Factors in Substance Abuse Treatment*, ed. S.L.A. Straussner. New York: Guilford Press, pp. 31-51.

Zeller, R.A. (1993), Combining qualitative and quantitative techniques to develop culturally sensitive measures. In: *Methodological Issues in AIDS Behavioral Research: AIDS Prevention and Mental Health*, eds. D.G. Ostrow & R.C. Kessler. New York: Plenum Press, pp. 95-116.

Evidence of HIV Transmission Risk in Barebacking Men-Who-Have-Sex-With-Men: Cases from the Internet

Alvin G. Dawson, Jr., MA
Michael W. Ross, PhD, MPH
Doug Henry, PhD
Anne Freeman, MSPH

SUMMARY. The purpose of this ethnographic study was to conduct an exploratory research investigation examining the phenomenon of barebacking among men-who-have-sex-with-men (MSM) on the Internet. The researchers selected a case sample of 100 MSM advertisers on an Internet bareback sex site to assess HIV transmission risk as related to HIV serostatus, partner selection, and sexual risk-taking. The data suggest that while intentionally seeking to transmit or contract HIV was ex-

Alvin G. Dawson, Jr. and Anne Freeman are affiliated with the University of Texas Southwestern Medical Center, Community Prevention and Intervention Unit, 400 South Zang #520, Dallas, TX 75208.

Michael W. Ross is affiliated with the University of Texas, School of Public Health.

Doug Henry is affiliated with the University of North Texas, Department of Anthropology, P.O. Box 310409, Denton, TX 76203.

Address correspondence to: Dr. Michael W. Ross, WHO Center for Health Promotion and Prevention Research, University of Texas School of Public Health, P.O. Box 20036, Houston, TX 77225.

[Haworth co-indexing entry note]: "Evidence of HIV Transmission Risk in Barebacking Men-Who-Have-Sex-With-Men: Cases from the Internet." Dawson, Alvin G., Jr. et al. Co-published simultaneously in *Journal of Gay & Lesbian Psychotherapy* (The Haworth Medical Press, an imprint of The Haworth Press, Inc.) Vol. 9, No. 3/4, 2005, pp. 73-83; and: *Barebacking: Psychosocial and Public Health Approaches* (ed: Perry N. Halkitis, Leo Wilton, and Jack Drescher) The Haworth Medical Press, an imprint of The Haworth Press, Inc., 2005, pp. 73-83. Single or multiple copies of this article are available for a fee from The Haworth Document Delivery Service [1-800-HAWORTH, 9:00 a.m. - 5:00 p.m. (EST). E-mail address: docdelivery@haworthpress.com].

Available online at http://www.haworthpress.com/web/JGLP
doi:10.1300/J236v09n03_05

tremely rare, a small proportion of advertisers appeared to be relatively indifferent to HIV transmission. However, the great majority of advertisers for bareback sex appeared to practice "sero-sorting" or sero-concordant behavior by HIV status with potential sexual partners as a strategy to minimize HIV transmission risk. *[Article copies available for a fee from The Haworth Document Delivery Service: 1-800-HAWORTH. E-mail address: <docdelivery@haworthpress.com> Website: <http://www.HaworthPress. com> © 2005 by The Haworth Press, Inc. All rights reserved.]*

KEYWORDS. AIDS, anal sex, barebacking, bisexual men, gay men, HIV, homosexuality, Internet, men-who-have-sex-with-men (MSM), safer sex, seroconcordant, serodiscordant, sero-sorting, STI

INTRODUCTION

The debate over "barebacking" among men-who-have-sex-with-men (MSM) has involved a considerable amount of contention, which often has been based on few empirical investigations (Mansergh et al., 2002; Halkitis, Parsons and Wilton, 2003; Halkitis et al., 2005). As noted in Gauthier and Forsyth's (1999) work, it is unclear as to whether the practice of bareback sex is actually on the rise, or if increased discussions concerning this phenomenon are fueling the controversy. Apart from often anecdotal or isolated cases cited in the media, there have been few studies that have investigated the levels of risk involved in barebacking, particularly as related to the use of the Internet. Much of the debate regarding barebacking has focused on deliberate transmission from an HIV infected to an uninfected person–often called "gift-giving" on the part of the donor and "bug-chasing" on the part of the recipient of the semen. Anecdotal evidence of this "eroticization" of HIV and the role it may play in increased incidence of unprotected anal intercourse (UAI) is noted by Suarez and Miller (2001). However, no empirical evidence exists either to support or disprove the existence, let alone the prevalence, of this phenomenon.

Historically, a rallying cry in the early eighties was the necessity for safer sex. The gay community banded together, braced with the evidence that UAI posed the greatest risk of HIV seroconversion. Various prevention strategies and programs aimed at curtailing the further spread of HIV disease were implemented. The impact of new and innovative treatments to combat HIV and its effect on the gay community can be seen on several levels (Carballo-Dieguez, 2001; Dilley, Woods and McFarland, 1997). However, complacency regarding safer sexual practices emerged in the gay community, particularly among those who had been severely affected by the loss of friends and loved ones (Ostrow et al., 2002). Others were virtually untouched by the physical and emotional impact of the disease. Consequently, some individuals perceived the contraction of HIV as inevitable. Others, falsely assured of their ability to outlast the disease due to newer drug therapies, began the return to condomless sex.

In the present era of HIV disease, the Internet has had an enormous impact on the way individuals in society interact with one another. Virtual communication has increasingly become a preferred method of interaction for many individuals. In the MSM community, the Internet has changed the rules of engagement in negotiations of sexual interaction. First and foremost, the capacity to seek out others willing to engage in barebacking activities has been facilitated by the Internet. Through e-mail, the World Wide Web, file transfer programs, Listservs and Internet Relay Chat, MSM may both advertise for and seek out like-minded individuals for condomless sex. For example, a variety of websites devoted to the phenomenon of barebacking identify the specific sexual activities in which they desire to participate, along with the preferred HIV serostatus of any perspective partners (Halkitis and Parsons, 2003; Bull, McFarlane and Rietmeijer, 2001; Gauthier and Forsyth, 1999).

SCOPE AND PREVALENCE OF THE BAREBACKING PHENOMENON

Mansergh et al. (2002) define barebacking as a socio-cultural phenomenon of intentional anal sex without a condom with someone other than a primary partner for various reasons or motivations. Mansergh differentiates deliberate barebacking from poor planning or spontaneous decisions about condom use. Recent reports in major cities across the United States (U.S.) report an increased incidence of sexually transmitted infections (STIs) such as syphilis, gonorrhea, Chlamydia, and hepatitis. Increases in STIs (other than HIV) suggest an increased incidence of unprotected anal intercourse (UAI) within the MSM community (Carballo-Dieguez, 2001). Mansergh et al. (2002) found that more than two-thirds of a sample of the 554 MSM had heard of the term "barebacking." Of particular interest was a discernible pattern of serostatus-sorting behavior, such as the tendency for HIV positive men to seek out other HIV positive men and HIV negative men to connect with HIV negative men for barebacking. The intent of this sero-sorting appears to be an effort to minimize HIV transmission risk and infection between men engaging in UAI. This interpretation appears to be supported by the observation that a greater number of HIV positive (as compared to HIV negative) men had engaged in unprotected receptive anal intercourse with an HIV positive partner. At the same time, a greater number of HIV negative (as compared to HIV positive) men reported UAI with HIV negative men (Suarez and Miller, 2001).

MOTIVATIONS FOR BAREBACKING

The barebacking phenomenon has initiated new tensions in the gay community as those who engage in this form of sexual expression have moved from the periphery of the community to claim a more visible role. Like Mansergh et al. (2002), Yep et al. (2002) have also noted the intentional aspect of bareback sex–stating that participation in unsafe sex may not be as simple as a singular occurrence of relapse into UAI. That there is an intentional pattern of risky behavior is further supported by the appearance of websites, personal ads, and gatherings devoted to bareback sex. In other words, for an unknown number of individuals, participation in condom-less sexual behavior is both intentional and negotiated (Carballo-Dieguez, 2001; Scarce, 1999).

Motivational triggers for barebacking include a view of safer sex as devoid of intimacy, detached, and lacking emotion while condomless sex is seen as a facilitator of connectedness. For seropositive MSM experiencing isolation, low self worth, and lack of appeal, intentional UAI may be used as a means of placating these more complex needs and desires (Gauthier and Forsyth, 1999; Gendin, 1997). Some who intentionally practice UAI say it fosters a sense of trust, belonging, and a shared "oneness" among those participating in this high-risk behavior. Illicit drug use to cope with stress may further increase the practice of UAI (Benotsch, Kalichman and Kelly, 1999; Halkitis and Parsons, 2002; Halkitis, Parsons and Wilton, 2003; McKirnan et al., 1996).

Complex motivations and situational factors, along with evolving community norms, may play a part in the decision of some MSM to participate in bareback sex. Carballo-Dieguez (2001) presents an overview of several facets affecting sexual behavior in four MSM over the course of approximately 20 years. The study's observations about the HIV epidemic identified attitudes that predicted future participation in barebacking behavior. Specifically addressing these findings will be important to the development and implementation of behavioral interventions targeting this high risk sexual activity (Suarez and Miller, 2001). However, although these observations provide a starting point for further exploration of the cultural and psychosocial issues surrounding barebacking, they may not be representative of views and behaviors of MSM in general, nor specifically of those who choose to participate in bareback activities.

BAREBACK SEX AND IDENTITY FORMATION

The construct of identity formation may be a useful means to provide insight into motivations for engaging in bareback sexual behaviors. Yep, Lovass and Pagonis (2002) present a conceptual framework to examine theoretical speculations as to how identity is formed. As in the larger society, labels are commonly used to differentiate oneself and groups of individuals within the MSM community. For some, one such identity is the "sexual adventurer" or "sexual outlaw" who explicitly engages in condomless anal intercourse. Such an identity deliberately violates the taboo of unsafe sex within the larger gay culture. In other words, barebacking may be seen as a way for some MSM to oppositionally construct a specific identity for themselves within the socio-cultural milieu of the wider gay community (Gendin, 1999).

Yep et al. (2002) further expanded on the conceptual definition and scope of barebacking behavior. They theorized that barebacking may be viewed as part of a "sexual outlaw" identity which is both resistant to behavioral norms imposed by either the gay community or society in general. This assertion is also echoed by the research of Gauthier and Forsyth (1999). They contend that the bareback phenomenon may serve as a marker of a cultural shift within the MSM community that redefines the boundaries of sexual behavior and personal identity. In pushing the boundaries of safer sexual practice further than is generally accepted within the gay community at large, individuals who bareback appear to be more sexually adventurous and seek higher levels of sensation (Carballo-Diequez, 2001).

The primary objective of this study was to conduct an ethnographic research investigation utilizing the Internet to examine the phenomenon of barebacking among MSM who frequented a bareback website from the Southwest region of the U.S.

METHODS

In March 2002, the authors accessed Barebackcity.com and extracted information on every fourth case from the Dallas zip code (75201) search, for the first 100 cases located up to eight miles from the central city. It was noted (where the information was provided) if there was a photograph included, sexual position preference (top, bottom, versatile), age, height, weight, HIV serostatus (positive, negative, no response [NR]), partner preferred status (positive, negative, no preference, NR), activity desired (one-on-one, three-way, groups/party/orgy/gang-bang, activity partner, long-term relationship), sexual activity preferred (insertive/receptive anal ejaculation; insertive, receptive oral ejaculation), bisexual interactions, have tattoos, piercings, and drug-friendly (all yes, no, NR).

The study compared the reported HIV serostatus of cases with partners' preferred serostatus, including those with no preference or no response, first in the seronegative followed by the seropositive categories. Comparison of the remaining variables was by HIV status and HIV status preferred in partners, sexual activities preferred, and those with stated HIV serostatus versus no mention of serostatus. Data analysis used SPSS version 12.0 with Chi-Squared tests with Yates correction for discontinuity for categorical variables and *t*-tests for the continuous variables. Significance was set at $p < .1$ due to the small sample and the pilot nature of the research.

RESULTS

Data were recorded on 100 cases. First, a "worst case" scenario was calculated. Here, cases whose HIV status was reported as either "no answer" or "positive" were all considered as HIV positive. These were compared by preferred partner serostatus (where "no preference" included a possibility for serodiscordant mixing). In this "worst case" scenario, three seropositive respondents preferred negative or "no preference" partners and 20 negative respondents preferred positive or had no preference for serostatus of partners. Thus, up to 23% of these cases may potentially be at risk for HIV transmission.

In a "best case" scenario, where all the HIV status "no answer" respondents were considered as seronegative, and those with "no preference" for serostatus of partner as preferring HIV negative partners, only one HIV positive respondent preferred negative partners, and no HIV negative respondents preferred positive partners. Thus, as few as one-percent may be at risk for HIV transmission.

Where sexual activities were contrasted by the reported HIV status of the case, there were no significant differences (insertive anal sex with ejaculation, $\chi^2 = 5.2$, ns; receptive anal sex with ejaculation, $\chi^2 = 6.3$, ns; insertive oral sex with ejaculation, $\chi^2 = 2.2$, ns; receptive oral sex with ejaculation, $\chi^2 = 5.6$, ns; all df = 4). Further, there were no significant differences by HIV status of the preferred partner (insertive anal sex with ejaculation, $\chi^2 = 3.7$, ns; receptive anal sex with ejaculation, $\chi^2 = 2.6$, ns; insertive oral sex with ejaculation, $\chi^2 = 1.1$, ns; receptive oral sex with ejaculation, $\chi^2 = 12.2$, ns; all df = 4).

Comparing those who had a specific preference for the HIV serostatus of partner (positive or negative) versus those with no preference, there was a non-significant trend for those with no preference for serostatus to be older (37.1 ± 6.8 vs. 34.4 ± 8.0 years, $t = 1.81$, df = 98, $p = .07$) and to be more likely to receive ejaculate orally (81% vs. 62%, $\chi^2 = 5.6$, df = 2, $p = .06$). HIV seropositive (versus seronegative) cases were significantly more likely to be older (38.1 ± 7.9 years, df = 80, $t = 2.1$, $p = .04$) and drug-friendly (50% vs. 28%, $\chi^2 = 15.2$, df = 6, $p = .02$).

DISCUSSION

Despite the relatively small sample, these data offer an interesting set of hypotheses about the barebacking phenomenon as seen through the lens of an Internet barebacking site. Of particular interest is the fact that in a "best case" scenario, where only known HIV status and specified HIV status of partner were used, no HIV negative cases wanted positive partners, and only one HIV positive case advertised for a negative partner. Thus, "gift giving" in this sample appeared to be very rare and "bug-chasing" was not represented at all. We conclude from these "best case" data that Internet cases who advertise for bareback sex do not appear to manifest the level of overt or intentional seeking for opportunities for HIV transmission that some media has suggested.

On the other hand, when those who provided no answer to HIV serostatus were considered to be seropositive while those with "no preference" for serostatus of partner were considered to include serodiscordant interactions, the level of potential risk rose to 23% of the sample. These data suggest that reported overt, deliberate potential for transmission of HIV is an extremely rare event; a level of reported indifference appears to be more common, although not the norm. There may be a perception that it is socially and legally safer to indicate "no preference" for HIV status of a partner than to specify a clearer openness to transmitting HIV. Nevertheless, in a "worst-case scenario," the less than a quarter of the sample might be at risk further suggests that avoidance of HIV transmission is the intention in the great majority of these cases. For those represented in these data, barebacking appears to be an activity undertaken with some consideration towards harm reduction. It could be compared, for the majority of cases, to be the equivalent of negotiated (although probably not verified) safety.

One further caveat is that it may be a leap of faith to equate an advertiser's report of their HIV status with their actual serostatus. It is not uncommon to have misrepresentation in Internet profiles, especially when the aim is to attract a sexual partner. Ross, Tikkanen and Manson (2000) note that misrepresentation in such circumstances may include (1) not mentioning potentially negative characteristics, (2) altering physical characteristics and age in a more flattering direction, (3) deliberate deception such as changing gender and race/ethnicity, and (4) posting a false or outdated picture. The lack of a verifiable identity on the Internet (and indeed the possibility that one individual may be the source of multiple identities) makes it difficult to assert with a high degree of confidence regarding the "truth" of personal data.

It is of particular interest that the sexual acts associated with HIV transmission, insertive and receptive anal and oral sex with ejaculation (by definition, in a barebacking sample, unprotected), were not significantly associated with HIV status of the case or the preferred partner's HIV status. This did not vary by acknowledged high risk activities (anal sex) or oral sex, the latter frequently perceived as lower risk activity. These data suggest that "sero-sorting" as a basis for risk management in this barebacking case sample is achieved by selecting seroconcordant partners. For example, whether the case considered himself a "top" or "bottom," as anticipated, was significantly associated with sexual activities preferred (insertive or receptive anal sex), indicating a degree of reliability in these findings.

These data support previous speculation in the research. For example, the level of indifference to transmission illustrated in the "worst case" scenario supports Mansergh et al.'s (2002) view that barebacking may be more likely due to poor planning rather than a deliberate intention to the possibility of transmission of HIV. These data also support Carballo-Dieguez's (2001) suggestion that serostatus assortative mixing (referred to here as "sero-sorting") is a major strategy for risk reduction by barebackers. The existence of organized barebacking sites, like the one studied here, supports Yep et al.'s (2002) contention that a specific barebacking identity appears to have emerged. However, this study provides no information about the prevalence of this phenomenon.

From a public health perspective, it is also important to note that even if "sero-sorting" behavior is used as a strategy to prevent HIV transmission, it has other adverse consequences. STIs such as syphilis, gonorrhea, hepatitis B, and herpes may be transmitted both anally and orally, and there is the possibility of transmission of different strains of HIV including drug-resistant ones (Holmes et al., 1999). Too narrow a focus on HIV underestimates the potential public health impact of HIV "sero-sorting," as recent epidemics of syphilis among MSM in major cities have demonstrated.

Finally, these data are subject to several limitations. Bias associated with self-report of risk cannot be estimated but may reflect an underestimation. This is especially likely given the potential legal implications of admitting one's intention to transmit a potentially fatal pathogen in a relatively conservative southern state. Further, these data were collected just prior to the 2003 U.S. Supreme Court *Lawrence v. Texas* case which lead to the decriminalization of homosexual behavior between adults in Texas and elsewhere. This decision may have influenced the risk-taking behavior of the individuals in the case sample. Further, this was an exploratory investigation on a relatively small sample, and there may also be biases in terms of region that suggest caution in generalizing these data to other areas in the United States.

CONCLUSIONS

These data suggest that the large majority of cases advertising for bareback sex, even in a worst-case scenario, involve assortative serostatus interactions and are specifically designed to minimize HIV transmission. Only in one case was a clear preference by a HIV positive individual for an HIV negative individual expressed. We conclude, on the face of these data, that the level of deliberate HIV transmission ("gift giving" or "bug chasing") in barebacking within this sample is extremely low, although the potential for indifferent transmission is unacceptably high. Research that focuses on those who express no desire for a partner of a particular serostatus, and their strategies for partner selection, is needed to answer the question as to the potential impact of HIV transmission in this group. These data suggest that the strategy of negotiating safety, or rather negotiating a *perception* of safety, by "serosorting" (based on accepting at face value the partners' self-belief of their serostatus) is the preferred method of prevention for HIV transmission. The relatively high level of lack of specification of HIV status preference has the effect of making *indifferent* transmission likely, rather than *deliberate* transmission. However, for the purposes of assessing public health risk, deliberate versus indifferent transmission may not vary much in their outcomes. These data also suggest that HIV "serosorting" is becoming a new version of the application of "folk epidemiology" (applying what defines degree of risk at the population level and what is known generally about the disease and its probability of transmission, to an individual level) about HIV prevention among gay men (Lowy and Ross, 1994). Perhaps, it is this indifference, subconscious rather than conscious HIV transmission, that needs to be targeted in HIV prevention in MSM populations.

REFERENCES

Benotsch, E.G., Kalichman, S.C. & Kelly, J.A. (1999), Sexual compulsivity and substance use in HIV-seropositive men who have sex with men: Prevalence and predictors of high risk sexual behaviors. *Addictive Behaviors*, 24:857-868.

Bull, S.S., McFarlane, M. & Rietmeijer, C. (2001), HIV and sexually transmitted infection risk behaviors among men seeking sex with men on-line. *American J. Public Health*, 91:988-989.

Carballo-Dieguez, A. (2001), HIV, barebacking, and gay men's sexuality, circa 2001. *J. Sex Education & Therapy*, 26:225-233.

Dilley, J.W., Woods, W.J. & McFarland, W. (1997), Are advances in treatment changing view about high-risk sex? *New England J. Medicine*, 337:501-502.

Gauthier D.K. & Forsyth, C. J. (1999), Bareback sex, bug chasers, and the gift of death. *Deviant Behavior*, 20:85-100.

Gendin, S. (1997), Riding bareback: Skin-on skin sex been there, done that, want more. *POZ Magazine*, pp. 64-65, June.

Gendin, S. (1999), They shoot barebackers, don't they? *POZ Magazine*, pp. 51-58, February.

Halkitis, P.N. & Parsons, J.T. (2002), Recreational drug use and HIV risk sexual behavior among men frequenting urban gay venues. *J. Gay & Lesbian Social Services*, 14:19-38.

Halkitis, P.N. & Parsons, J.T. (2003), Intentional unsafe sex (barebacking) among men who meet sexual partners on the Internet. *AIDS Care*, 15:367-378.

Halkitis, P.N., Parsons, J.T. & Wilton. L. (2003), Barebacking among gay and bisexual men in New York City: Explanations for the emergence of intentional unsafe behavior. *Archives Sexual Behavior*, 32:351-358.

Halkitis, P.N., Parsons, J.T. & Wilton, L. (2003), An exploratory study of contextual and situational factors related to methamphetamine use among gay and bisexual men in New York City. *J. Drug Issues*, 33:413-432.

Halkitis, P.N., Wilton, L., Parsons, J.T. & Hoff, C. (2004), Correlates of sexual risk-taking behavior among HIV seropositive gay men in seroconcordant primary partner relationships. *Psychology, Health, & Medicine*, 9:99-113.

Halkitis, P.N., Wilton, L., Wolitski, R., Parsons, J.T , Hoff, C. & Bimbi, D. (2005), Barebacking identity among HIV-positive gay and bisexual men: Demographic, psychological, and behavior correlates. *AIDS*(Suppl): 527-535.

Holmes, K.K., Mårdh, P.A., Sparling, P.F., Lemon, S.M., Stamm, W.E., Piot, P. & Wasserheit, J.N., eds. (1999), *Sexually Transmitted Diseases (3rd Edition)*, New York: McGraw-Hill.

Lowy, E. & Ross, M.W. (1994), "It'll never happen to me": Gay men's beliefs, perceptions and folk constructions of sexual risk. *AIDS Education & Prevention*, 6:467-482.

Mansergh, G., Marks, G., Colfax, G.N., Guzman, R., Rader, M. & Buchbinder, S. (2002), "Barebacking" in a diverse sample of men who have sex with men. *AIDS*, 16:653-659.

McKirnan, D.J., Ostrow, D.G. & Hope, B. (1996), Sex, drugs and escape: A psychological model of HIV-risk sexual behaviours. *AIDS Care*, 8:655-669.

Ostrow, D.E., Fox, K.J., Chmiel, J.S., Silvestre, A., Bisscher, B.R., Vanable, P.A., Jacobson, L.P. et al. (2002), Attitudes towards highly active antiretroviral therapy are associated with sexual risk taking among HIV-infected and uninfected homosexual men. *AIDS*, 16:775-780.

Ross M.W., Tikkanen, R. & Mansson, S.A. (2000), Differences between Internet samples and conventional samples of men who have sex with men: Implications for research and HIV interventions. *Social Science & Medicine*, 51:749-758.

Scarce, M. (1999), A ride on the wild side. *POZ Magazine*, pp. 52-55, 70-71, February.

Suarez, T. & Miller, J. (2001), Negotiating risks in context: A perspective on unprotected anal intercourse and barebacking among men who have sex with men: Where do we go from here? *Archives Sexual Behavior*, 30:287-300.

Yep, G.A., Lovass, K & Pagonis, A.V. (2002), The case of "riding bareback": Sexual practices and the paradoxes of identity in the era of AIDS. *J. Homosexuality*, 42:1-14.

Barebacking Among Internet Based Male Sex Workers

David S. Bimbi, MA
Jeffrey T. Parsons, PhD

SUMMARY. Some have raised concern that male sex workers (MSWs) serve as "vectors of transmission" of HIV into the heterosexual community. Research on MSWs, however, has found that these men report unsafe sex more often with casual partners than with clients. In the mid-1990s, two new phenomena emerged: the Internet, providing a new way for MSWs to meet clients, and barebacking or intentional anal sex without condoms. Using qualitative and quantitative methods in an effort to understand the impact of these phenomena, this study sought to explore intentions for unsafe sex among MSWs who reach clients through the Internet. Findings suggest that most MSWs do not intentionally seek out sex without condoms or engage in barebacking. This does not denote the complete absence of sexual

David S. Bimbi is affiliated with the Center for HIV/AIDS Educational Studies and Training (CHEST) and the Graduate Center, City University of New York.

Jeffrey T. Parsons is affiliated with the Center for HIV/AIDS Educational Studies and Training (CHEST), the Graduate Center and Hunter College, City University of New York.

Address correspondence to: Jeffrey T. Parsons, Hunter College, 695 Park Avenue, New York, NY 10021 (E-mail: jeffrey.parsons@hunter.cuny.edu).

The authors would like to thank Jose Nanin for his assistance in the preparation of this manuscript as well as James Kelleher and the other members of the Center for HIV/AIDS Educational Studies and Training (CHEST) team for their assistance and support with this project. The authors would also like to thank the participants and the members of the community who encouraged them to undertake this investigation.

[Haworth co-indexing entry note]: "Barebacking Among Internet Based Male Sex Workers." Bimbi, David S. and Jeffrey T. Parsons. Co-published simultaneously in *Journal of Gay & Lesbian Psychotherapy* (The Haworth Medical Press, an imprint of The Haworth Press, Inc.) Vol. 9, No. 3/4, 2005, pp. 85-105; and: *Barebacking: Psychosocial and Public Health Approaches* (ed: Perry N. Halkitis, Leo Wilton, and Jack Drescher) The Haworth Medical Press, an imprint of The Haworth Press, Inc., 2005, pp. 85-105. Single or multiple copies of this article are available for a fee from The Haworth Document Delivery Service [1-800-HAWORTH, 9:00 a.m. - 5:00 p.m. (EST). E-mail address: docdelivery@haworthpress.com].

risk behaviors, particularly with casual partners as found in previous research. Interview data suggest that these men may be employing harm reduction strategies such as partner characteristics and sex role positioning in
their decision making processes. These findings can be helpful to service
providers who currently or plan to provide intervention services to members
of this population. *[Article copies available for a fee from The Haworth Document Delivery Service: 1-800-HAWORTH. E-mail address: <docdelivery@
haworthpress.com> Website: <http://www.HaworthPress.com> © 2005 by The
Haworth Press, Inc. All rights reserved.]*

KEYWORDS. AIDS, anal sex, barebacking, condoms, gay men, harm
reduction, HIV, homosexuality, male sex workers, MSW, prostitution,
safer sex, sex workers, STI

Since early in the AIDS epidemic, some research has suggested that
the heterosexual community is more at risk of contracting HIV from
male sex workers (MSWs) through clients (who are married heterosexual men) as compared to men in the gay community (Coutinho,
van Andel and Rijsdijk, 1988). In a widely cited article, Morse and
his colleagues (1991) portrayed male sex workers (MSWs) as "vectors of transmission" of HIV into heterosexual society employing the
same argument. It is unclear, however, from Morse et al.'s data
whether the anal sex behaviors reported in their sample occurred
with or without condoms. A growing body of evidence published in
the 1990s directly questions the assertion that MSWs are engaging in
unsafe anal sex with clients and spreading HIV into the heterosexual
community (Browne and Minichiello, 1996; Estcourt et al., 2000;
Estep, Waldorf and Marotta, 1992; Hickson et al., 1994; Minichiello
et al., 2000; Minichiello et al., 2001; Overs, 1991; Parsons, Bimbi
and Halkitis, 2001; Perkins et al., 1993; Pleak and Meyer-Bahlburg,
1990; Ziersch, Gaffney and Tomlinson, 2000). These studies report
that MSWs use condoms more consistently with clients than they do
with casual (non-paying) male partners. Therefore, it appears that
casual partners are more at risk of contracting HIV and sexually
transmitted infections (STIs) from MSWs than are the clients of
these men.

This risk to casual partners is supported by epidemiological data published since the mid-1990s, which suggests an alarming increase in unprotected sexual behaviors among gay and bisexual men in urban areas

with visible gay communities (Chen et al., 2002; Wolitski et al., 2001). The mainstream gay press (Agosto, 2001; Gallagher, 1998; Ocamb, 1999; Savage, 1999; Signorile, 1998) as well as magazines aimed at an HIV-positive readership (Gendin, 1999; Scarce, 1999; Warner, 1997) have tried to explain this increase. Some researchers suggest that gay men have become tired of condoms and safer sex messages (Wolitski et al., 2001). Others argue that some gay men are deliberately looking for unsafe sex. The intentional pursuit of unprotected sex has led to the development of a new vernacular, with terms like *barebacking*, *raw*, and *skin to skin* (Gendin, 1997).

Efforts to explain this phenomena among HIV-positive gay men have faulted the "AIDS establishment's" safer sex education campaigns. These campaigns have been criticized for sidestepping the altruistic concern of preventing viral transmission to others and instead focusing on reminding HIV-positive men that they may be putting themselves at risk for opportunistic infections or re-infection with a different strain of HIV (Rotello, 1997, p. 109). Even academics have taken note of the barebacking phenomenon and have tried to explain it from the perspectives of sociology (Gauthier and Forsyth, 1999), anthropology (Junge, 2002), psychology (Mansergh et al., 2002; Suarez and Miller, 2001), and queer theory (Yep, Lovaas and Pagonis, 2002). Each of these perspectives defines "barebacking" as intentional anal sex without a condom.[1]

Though it has emerged as a salient issue in the gay press and recently in the academic literature, few researchers have explicitly addressed barebacking within the context of sex work. Nor has the issue of how barebacking behavior may vary across the venues in which MSWs meet their potential clients been specifically addressed.

Typically, in Western nations, venues for MSWs consist of three types: *direct* client-to-customer contact on the streets or in bars, *mediated* contact through an escort agency, and *passive* contact through the use of advertisements. Researchers have created a nomenclature for different types of MSWs based on the venue of contact (Allen, 1980; Caulkins and Coombs, 1976; Weisberg, 1985), although it should be noted that these terms often are used interchangeably. *Hustlers* actively seek out clients on the streets or in bars. Some research suggests hustlers are more likely to self-identify as heterosexual, and provide sexual services (usually limited to insertive oral or anal sex) to men as a means of obtaining money or drugs (Calhoun and Weaver, 1996). *Call boys* are men with whom potential clients make direct contact by telephone (Allen, 1980) or through a third party that acts as an intermediary and charges a "commission." *Escorts* are usually gay and bisexually identified men who advertise in gay publications (Hickson et al., 1994; Lumby, 1978; Parsons, Bimbi and Halkitis, 2001; Salamon, 1989). Finally, younger men who are financially and materially supported by an older man in exchange for sexual contact are called *kept boys* (Bloor, McKeganey and Barnard, 1990; West and de Villiers, 1993).

Since the late 1960s, agencies providing MSWs for men have been in operation (Salamon, 1989) and individual escorts have been advertising their services as models, masseurs, body workers, or escorts in gay magazines and newspapers (Lumby, 1978). With the growing popular use of the Internet, a new venue for advertisements has emerged as well. Many escorts maintain their own websites, which often include photos and descriptions of their services. Potential clients are able to locate escorts on the Internet through their individual websites, "escort finder" websites or in popular Internet chat rooms. However, some Internet service providers have banned the use of the word "escort" in user profiles and in user created chat rooms.

It is important to note that most research concerning the psychosocial and physical health of MSWs has focused on hustlers (Hickson et al., 1994). However, Internet-based escorts may differ substantially from other types of MSWs. Whereas hustlers risk arrest, potential for violence, and not being paid for services rendered–perhaps due to the fact that they market themselves on the street–these problems may be less likely to affect escorts (Calhoun and Weaver, 1996).

Researchers have recently begun to make efforts to include a wider range of MSWs in their investigations. They have reported that escorts are more likely to engage in a several different sexual activities with a client during a single meeting than other types of MSWs (Minichiello et al., 2000). It is therefore possible that HIV risk behaviors among escorts may differ from those of other MSWs. For example, Internet-based escorts have the ability to negotiate safer sex on-line and reduce the potential risk of rejection by a client at the arranged meeting time. Escorts can be more selective about their clients, charge more for their services, and have greater control of their work schedule.

The focus of the present study is to ascertain whether Internet-based male escorts are contributing to the transmission of HIV by determining if they are intentionally having condomless anal sex (barebacking) with clients and casual sexual partners.

METHOD

Procedure

The e-mail addresses of potential participants were identified through America Online user profiles and various male escort websites. An e-mail inviting the men to telephone and be screened for the study was sent to 370 valid e-mail addresses. The e-mail invitation assured potential participants of the confidential nature of the research study, which was approved by the Institutional Review Board of the authors, as well as a disclaimer of any link to law enforcement agencies. Eligibility criteria included self-identification as a gay or bisexual male, self-reported sex work in the past 90 days, and age 18 or older.

A total of 60 phone calls were received, and 57 men were screened and eligible for the study. Out of this number, 50 men presented for the study. Participants provided informed consent and were then interviewed by trained male staff. Interviews were audiotaped and lasted up to 75 minutes. The audiotapes were sent to an independent firm for transcription and reviewed by the authors to remove any identifying information to maintain participant confidentiality. Following the interview, the participants completed a self-administered quantitative survey. Participants were offered 75 dollars for their time and effort.

Measures

Sociodemographics. Participants were asked their age, race/ethnicity, employment status, income, education, HIV status, sexual orientation and if they had a primary partner. Additionally, participants were asked how long they had worked as an escort and the time spent each week devoted to sex-work related activities including communicating with potential clients or time spent traveling.

Sexual Behaviors. Participants were asked to indicate the frequency of sexual risk behaviors in the three months prior to completion of the survey with both work-related and non-work related sexual partners of unknown HIV status.

Barebacking Intentions. This scale consisted of four items, reflecting insertive and receptive oral and anal sex behaviors written specifically for this study. Each item was preceded by the statement "I purposely seek out____" followed by the risk behavior (bareback sex as a top, guys who will let me eat their cum, etc.). Participants rated each item from 1 to 5 with strongly disagree and strongly agree as anchor points. Cronbach's alpha for the four item scale was .70.

Qualitative Interview

The questions were asked in a semi-structured format that encouraged participants to elaborate on their thoughts, feelings, and experiences. The interview protocol focused on a variety of areas, including limits and boundaries for sex work (i.e., barebacking unsafe sex, sexual practices, etc.) as well as detailed narratives of their most recent sexual experiences with clients and non-paying partners (which could be either their current primary partner or a casual partner).

Analytic Strategy

Quantitative data was analyzed using SPSS version 12. Qualitative interviews were organized utilizing QSR NUD-IST software which permitted statements regarding barebacking to be identified and then organized into common themes identified by the authors. Excerpts from the interviews for this study will be accompanied by the participant's ID number as well as their age, ethnicity, and self-reported HIV status.

RESULTS

Results from the quantitative surveys are presented first, followed by illustrative quotes from the qualitative interviews. This sequence is intended to provide the reader with further insight into interpreting the survey results.

Participant Characteristics

Of the 50 men in the sample, most were white, young, gay-identified and HIV-negative (see Table 1). There were only two men who never had been tested for HIV due to their belief (stated in the qualitative interview) that it was unnecessary since they never engaged in receptive anal intercourse. Twenty-one of the participants (45.6%) reported a history of sexually transmitted infections (STIs) other than HIV, such as gonorrhea or syphilis. In the three months prior to assessment, the men reported engaging in sexual activity with an average of 30 ($SD = 35.85$)

TABLE 1. Participant demographics and health characteristics ($n = 50$)

	n	%
Sexual Orientation		
Homosexual/Gay	41	82.0%
Bisexual	9	18.0%
HIV status		
HIV negative	40	80.0%
HIV positive	8	16.0%
Untested	2	4.0%
Ethnicity		
African American	5	10.0%
Asian/Pacific Islander	3	6.0%
Caucasian	35	70.0%
Latino	7	14.0%
Education		
High School or Less	4	8.0%
Some College	14	30.0%
Bachelor's Degree	22	44.0%
Graduate Coursework/Degree	10	20.0%

work-related and 19 ($SD = 47.42$) non work-related sexual partners of unknown HIV status.

None of the bisexually-identified men reported sex with women in the previous three months nor did any have a female primary partner. A total of 17 men (34%) did report having a male primary partner. The median income range reported from sources other than sex work was $10,000 to $19,999. The median income range reported from sex work was $20,000 to $29,999. The average length of time the sample reported working as escorts was 2.66 years ($SD = 5.03$), with a range from 3 weeks to 25 years. About half of the men ($n = 23$) reported spending at least 12 hours a week escorting or performing escorting-related activities (such as answering phone calls or communicating with potential clients online); 26% ($n = 12$) reported spending more than 20 hours a week escorting, and could be considered "full time" or nearly "full-time" sex workers. More than two-thirds of the men (70%, $n = 32$) charged $200 an hour, with a range from $75 for "body work" to $250 for "full service."

Quantitative Insights into Barebacking

In the paper-pencil survey portion of the interview, HIV-negative MSWs reported higher overall frequencies of all sexual risk behaviors with casual partners than with clients of unknown HIV status (Table 2). For example, 23.8% of the HIV-negative MSWs reported engaging in the behavior that places them most at risk for infection with HIV with casual partners: unprotected anal receptive sex with ejaculation. The reported frequency for the same behavior with clients was less, 11.9%. The HIV-positive MSWs in the sample reported higher percentages of sexual risk-taking that were almost consistent for both client and casual partner for all behaviors. Half of the HIV-positive MSWs reported engaging in unprotected anal insertive sex with ejaculation, regardless of partner type–the behavior most associated with HIV transmission. Unprotected, oral insertive sex with ejaculation was the most frequent behavior reported by both HIV-negative and HIV-positive MSWs in this sample across both partner types.

However, endorsement of intentions for sexual risk behaviors, indicated by the choices of "agree" or "strongly agree" as a response, was *not* as prevalent as were the reported frequencies of unsafe sex among both HIV-negative and HIV-positive MSWs (Table 3). In fact, there was only one individual among the HIV-positive MSWs who endorsed three out of four sexual risk behaviors. Endorsement of intentions for unprotected, oral insertive sex with ejaculation was highest among the HIV-negative MSWs in this sample.

The correlation between responses for intentions to engage in sexual risk behaviors with the actual frequencies of those risk behaviors, with both clients and casual partners of unknown HIV status, indicates a significant relationship does exist between some risk intentions and sexual behaviors (Table 4). However, due to the very low number of HIV-positive participants, the correlations reported should be viewed with caution; the findings may differ with a larger sample of these men. Among the HIV-negative MSWs, correlations between intentions and behaviors were significant for unprotected anal insertive sex with both clients and casual partners. Conversely, a significant relationship between intentions and reported behavior among HIV-positive MSWs was ob-

TABLE 2. Frequency of participants reporting any unprotected sexual behaviors with partners of unknown HIV status ($n = 50$)

HIV Negative/Untested MSWs ($n = 42$)				
	Work Partners		Casual Partners	
	(Mean = 25.95, range 1-150)		(Mean = 11.46, range 0-40)	
	n	%	n	%
Anal Receptive, no ejaculation	5	11.9	10	23.8
Anal Receptive, w/ejaculation	1	2.3	5	11.9
Oral Receptive, w/ejaculation	6	14.3	8	19.0
Anal Insertive, no ejaculation	6	14.3	14	33.3
Anal Insertive, w/ejaculation	3	7.1	3	7.1
Oral Insertive, w/ejaculation	24	57.1	22	52.4

HIV Positive MSWs ($n = 8$)				
	Work Partners		Casual Partners	
	(Mean = 54.25, range 10-170)		(Mean = 62.29, range 0-325)	
	n	%	n	%
Anal Receptive, no ejaculation	4	50.0	2	25.0
Anal Receptive, w/ejaculation	2	25.0	4	50.0
Oral Receptive, w/ejaculation	4	50.0	4	50.0
Anal Insertive, no ejaculation	4	50.0	4	50.0
Anal Insertive, w/ejaculation	1	12.5	1	12.5
Oral Insertive, w/ejaculation	5	62.5	2	25.0

served with partners, regardless of type, for unprotected anal receptive sex with or without ejaculation. However among both HIV-negative and HIV-positive MSWs, the relationship between intentions and unprotected oral receptive sex with ejaculation was significant across both partner types.

Qualitative Insights Regarding Barebacking

None of the interview questions specifically asked participants to speak about barebacking. Nonetheless, most participants ($n = 40$, 87.0%) dis-

TABLE 3. Intentions for unprotected sex among male escorts ($n = 48$)

HIV Negative/Untested MSWs ($n = 41$)

	Strongly Agree/ Agree		Neither		Disagree/ Strongly Disagree	
	n	%	*n*	%	*n*	%
Anal Insertive	3	7.3	3	7.3%	35	85.4
Anal Receptive	3	7.3	3	7.3	35	85.4
Oral Insertive, w/ejaculation	4	9.7	9	22.0	28	68.3
Oral Receptive, w/ejaculation	1	2.4	6	14.6	34	83.0

HIV Positive MSWs ($n = 7$)

	Strongly Agree/ Agree		Neither		Disagree/ Strongly Disagree	
	n	%	*n*	%	*n*	%
Anal Insertive	0	0.0	0	0.0%	7	100.0
Anal Receptive	1	14.3	0	0.0	6	85.7
Oral Insertive, w/ejaculation	1	14.3	1	14.3	5	71.4
Oral Receptive, w/ejaculation	1	14.3	1	14.3	5	71.4

cussed barebacking during their qualitative interviews. Typically, barebacking was discussed in the context of limits that MSWs set with regard to sex work practices or in terms of describing interactions with clients.

From the accounts of MSWs, it appears that HIV risk is of little concern to some clients. Most men ($n = 37$, 80.0%) stated that they had clients request bareback sex on at least one occasion:[2]

> You get a lot of guys who don't want you to use condoms. They'll say, "I want you to fuck me without a condom and come inside me," or whatever. They just don't care. . . . guys are very unsafe . . .

TABLE 4. Correlations between intentions for sexual risk behaviors and frequency of unprotected sex acts with unknown HIV status partners in the prior three months among male escorts (*n* = 48)

HIV Negative/Untested MSWs (*n* = 41)				
	Behavior			
	Work Partners		Casual Partners	
BB as top	AIE = .556**	AIN = .025	AIE = .448**	AIN = .395*
BB as bottom	ARE = .439**	ARN = .503**	ARE = .025	ARN = .033
Give cum orally	OIE = .014		OIE = .052	
Take cum orally	ORE = .471**		ORE = .336*	

HIV Positive MSWs (*n* = 7)				
	Behavior			
	Work Partners		Casual Partners	
BB as top	AIE = −.167	AIN = .960**	AIE = −.167	AIN = .842*
BB as bottom	ARE = .997**	ARN = .637	ARE = 1.00**	ARN = .996**
Give cum orally	OIE = .366		OIE = .754	
Take cum orally	ORE = .844*		ORE = .834*	

* Significant at the 0.01 level, ** Significant at the 0.05 level

they're not going to get it from me, but there's going to be somebody out there who's going to come along and do this for them. (Age 46, White, HIV-negative)

If anybody asks me if . . . if I'll fuck them bareback, I'd say, I'd rather not. If they push it, then I just basically say there's some guys I can suggest to you, but I don't do that. (Age 40, White, HIV-negative)

Some guys want me to fuck them bareback, which I won't do. I just tell them I won't do that and see what happens. . . . Well, it doesn't happen very often, but times that it did, he says "that's okay," and "all right, I'll use a condom." There was another time when someone said "okay I'll find someone else." (Age 27, White, HIV-negative)

Sometimes requests for bareback sex are made up-front by clients–either by phone, e-mail, or instant messaging (IM)–before an appointment is scheduled:

> Oh, I lose a lot of clients because of that. I'd say maybe between thirty and forty percent. One guy keeps hounding me about it to the point where he wants to fly me to where he lives just for [bareback sex]. (Age 33, White, HIV-negative)

> I have an automatic answering machine on the computer, and when I get IMs, people generally come in and ask particular questions like rate, and barebacking will come up. And it's come up a lot lately. It seems like every other request is for barebacking these days. Seriously. (Age 39, White, HIV-negative)

It was less common for clients to request bareback sex in person, although there were some MSW reports of instances in which this happened:

> I've been in a few sexual situations where the clients have actually removed my condom and asked me to fuck them raw . . . with the prospect of paying a lot more money to do so . . . One guy said a thousand bucks if I fucked him raw. (Age 39, White, HIV-negative)

> I'm really shocked at how . . . how people are taking risks. I do get a lot of requests. Not a lot of requests through e-mail, but when I'm there doing it people will . . . I mean, unless I bring it up or get out the condom, they would just sit on my dick without even asking about it. (Age 36, White, HIV-positive)

Among the HIV-negative escorts, barebacking was typically viewed as too much of a risk. More than half of the men ($n = 30$; 65.2%) made it very clear that bareback sex was off-limits with clients.

> They wonder what you're doing. "You're a barebacker. You want me to pay extra for you not to wear a condom." I say "no" because [HIV is] forever, and I don't care how much money you got, it

won't last me forever. I don't want to be sick. That's all I got is my health. (Age 22, Latino, HIV-negative)

I asked him, "Should I bring the condoms?" And he said, "Oh, I thought we were doing BB," which at one point I didn't know what that was. And I was like, "What do you mean?" And he said, "I want us to do bareback." I'm like, "No, you got the wrong person. I'm sorry for wasting your time." (Age 26, Latino, HIV-negative)

I will always have safe sex and even if the client mentions something about unsafe sex, it's not going to happen. It's such a turn-off, I cannot sustain an erection like that. Because this person is unsafe. (Age 25, White, HIV-negative)

Even after being offered extra money for bareback sex, one escort reporting refusing:

I just excused myself. It was getting out of hand. I stopped the session. I left . . . The guy was really drugged up and . . . he wasn't going to be happy until he got what he wanted. (Age 39, White, HIV-negative)

A few men, however, described a willingness to have bareback sex with casual partners although not with their clients:

Usually the client feels the need to mention everything he likes, and I've had people say, "Oh, I like a guy to come in me," or whatever. For fun, I've only barebacked with people I know. You know, fuck-buddies, flings, whatever you want to call them. Otherwise, I'm safe. (Age 22, White, HIV-negative)

I have [barebacked] as a top a few times, but never as a bottom. And I don't think I will ever do that professionally. I mean, [maybe] if I were with a friend or with a boyfriend over a period of time. (Age 44, White, HIV-negative)

A willingness to engage in barebacking with casual sex partners was often associated with lower perceptions of risk. Some of the subjects perceived a reduced barebacking risk associated with certain contextual factors, for example, if the sexual act itself did not last a long time:

It kind of just happened. But usually I'm aware it's happening and I don't let it go on for that long . . . I know there's a risk. . . . but my mind is set . . , if I'm going to get something, I'm going to get it . . . You never can be a hundred percent safe. (Age 22, White, HIV-negative)

[Although I had been] having safe sex for twenty fucking years, after I went on-line, I barebacked three times. But when I say bareback, I don't mean I fucked them for an hour. I mean, I stuck my dick in them like for two or three minutes. . . . I couldn't believe I was doing it. And yet there was something so powerful about it. This one guy, it was a minute. There was another guy, it was two minutes, and with the third guy it was three minutes. I'm not talking about fucking to anywhere near pre-come or coming. I had to feel what an asshole felt like with my dick, because I'd been so fucking responsible for so goddamn long, I just couldn't take it anymore. (Age 42, White, HIV-negative)

A minority of subjects ($n = 9$; 19.6%) did admit to barebacking with clients. Most of these men expressed concern about such behavior, although a few reported that barebacking was their preferred type of sex with clients.

I even have been with clients that asked me to bareback. And I've done it. I'm not going to lie. I've done it, because I want them to enjoy it. But then afterwards, it's like, damn, I just did it. I don't know if I'm going to see this person again. I don't know what they have. I mean, I'm constantly tested, but what about them? So you can say it's safe, but the majority of the time we're really not playing it safe. (Age 27, African American, HIV-negative)

Just yesterday, I listed my site on Bareback Ring on the web. I know my hits are up over two hundred clients a day now because of it. But when people have asked about it, I sometimes say, "It depends on who I'm with." That's my standard answer. I find that's a safe answer, rather than "Yes, yes, yes," because you might be turning away somebody who is against it. People are testing you . . . The ones that particularly ask for bareback sex don't ask about health at all. It's not talked about. (Age 25, White, HIV-positive)

Again, the issue of perceived risk was a common theme. Of those who reported barebacking with clients, the HIV-negative men felt that they were "safer" from contracting HIV or STIs if they were the inserter.

> Everyone that I'm with, whether they tell me they're HIV positive or not, I assume is HIV positive; therefore, I choose to play safe. But, I can say I have barebacked before when I'm on top, because I don't think about the risk. Sometimes I'll negotiate barebacking a guy if he is on the bottom, but if I'm on the bottom, I always make them use a condom. (Age 23, African American, HIV-negative)

Some of the HIV-positive men, however, expressed the same views. That is, they reported a willingness to bareback as a top, but not as a bottom. These men assumed that those willing to bareback as a bottom must also be HIV-positive. They were not as worried about transmitting HIV to others, but instead were concerned about contracting a different strain of HIV:

> I don't really like to do barebacking. If they insist on it, I will, but I just don't think it's a safe thing to do. For my own safety I am selective doing that . . . I don't bareback on the bottom. I will bareback top, but again, that's their choice. But I let them know up front that I am positive when they want me to do that. So, you know, I'm advising them at the time. (Age 28, African American/White, HIV-positive)

> I don't want them coming inside of me. So that's what I tell them. If I bareback, I always tell them, "I'll let you, but don't you dare come inside me." I do tell them that. And a couple of times I've had guys who didn't listen. And I didn't get physical, but I almost did. (Age 30, White, HIV-positive)

Sometimes, subjects felt they were minimizing any potential risk from barebacking with clients. One man felt his clients had too much money to pose a risk to him with regard to his health:

> I don't think, that I would say, "I can't [bareback]" unless I had doubts about their having some other kind of STD. I'd rather not have crabs or gonorrhea. But, my rates are high enough to see people who have a certain income and a certain lifestyle and that, in

general, cushions me from those sorts of things. (Age 25, Asian/ Pacific Islander, HIV-negative)

Another participant felt that he was able to visually ascertain any potential risk by examining the genitals of his partners prior to barebacking:

> I've let guys inside me. Typically, before I let them in–I know this doesn't make any sense–but I actually will look at their dick and their balls, and I'll do an assessment to see if I see lesions or something. From my nursing background, I'm very good at determining what I see. And I've confronted guys and told them you should have yourself checked out because you have problems. And they get up and leave, and I don't care. (Age 30, White, HIV-positive)

Some subjects described being tempted to engage in bareback sex. Typically, the temptation revolved around the attractiveness of the potential sexual partner. When asked about the types of clients with whom he would be tempted to bareback, one participant said: "If he was just really hot–had a hot ass. I just gotta have it." (Age 31, White, HIV-negative). A similar sentiment was expressed by another participant:

> Right after I got on the Internet, I was having the most gorgeous fucking bottoms I could ever want . . . sending me their pictures, begging me to come over for me to fuck them. It was like a kid in a candy story. And a lot of them wanted to bareback, and my immediate reaction was no, no. If this guy is a barebacker, he's at risk for STDs. But when I finally started getting a couple of them over there and they were really beautiful, suddenly the desire to do it struck me once, twice, three times. But after the third time having done it, I pulled myself back and I said I don't want to . . . I don't want to let go . . . it felt right when I did this. I've been safe for twenty fucking years. It's all right that I stuck my dick in three different guys' asses for a total of five minutes. That's okay. But I don't want to get caught up in that. And I'm going to stop it. And I have. (Age 42, White, HIV-negative)

DISCUSSION

Regardless of reported differences in unsafe or risky sexual behaviors among partner types, the MSWs in this sample, both HIV-negative and HIV-positive, appear to engage in barebacking at similar rates as those reported in community samples of gay and bisexual men. Therefore, the Internet-based male escorts in our sample may more closely resemble other gay men as a whole, rather than other types of MSWs, such as hustlers working the streets for survival sex. However, as there were a very limited number of HIV-positive men in the sample, making definitive statements about this sub-sample would be inappropriate.

Supporting the results of numerous other studies, the participants were similar to other samples of MSWs, specifically those including men who describe themselves as "escorts" (Browne and Minichiello, 1995; Estcourt et al., 2000; Estep, Waldorf and Marotta, 1992; Hickson et al., 1994; Minichiello et al., 2000; Overs, 1991; Perkins et al., 1993; Pleak and Meyer-Bahlburg, 1990; Ziersch et al., 2000). The participants in this study reported higher overall instances of all sexual risk behaviors with casual partners than with clients with only one exception: unprotected oral insertive sex with ejaculation which is addressed below. Therefore, this study adds to a growing body of literature which challenges the assumption that MSWs, at least those calling themselves escorts, are a vector of transmission for infection among heterosexuals.

Furthermore, the significant correlations reported herein only demonstrate that participants who agreed with statements regarding intentions for sexual risk behaviors were the same persons reporting that they had engaged frequently in those behaviors. The frequencies of agreement reported clearly indicate that most of the sample is not intentionally seeking out sexual risk behaviors. If risky sex was reported, it may be due to factors other than barebacking and intentionally engaging in risky sex.

The qualitative findings clearly lend support to the above arguments. Most of the escorts in our sample reported turning down explicit requests for barebacking from clients. This does not imply that risk was not reported; in fact, the frequencies of any unsafe sex reported with clients and casual partners indicates that it was. However, the qualitative findings demonstrate that many of the men expressed ideas suggesting a willingness to engage in certain risk behaviors depending upon the situation and partner. This implies that these men may be informally utilizing harm reduction strategies.

Those HIV-negative men that did engage in unprotected receptive sex with clients may be doing so in the belief that they are less at risk with the latter than with other types of partners. For example, an HIV-negative man may believe he is less at risk engaging in unprotected anal receptive sex with a married client who identifies as heterosexual than with a casual gay partner he met in a bathhouse. The HIV-negative MSWs in our sample also reported in the interviews, strategies, valid or not, for judging the "safety" of engaging in unprotected anal sex with partners of either type.

Conversely, the HIV-positive men in the sample may be engaging in unsafe sex due to differential attitudes that HIV-positive men have about the risks of unsafe sex to themselves (Green, 1996; Gendin, 1997; Wolitski et al., 2001). Additionally, while the HIV-positive men report some willingness to engage in unprotected insertive sex as an inserter, they reported doing so to protect themselves by avoiding re-infection with other strains of HIV and infection with other STIs. While some HIV-positive escorts stated a belief that any person willing to engage in unprotected anal receptive sex must also be HIV-positive, only one of the eight HIV-positive participants reported ejaculating inside a partner. The HIV-positive MSW may engage in unprotected anal insertive sex with men he assumes to be HIV-positive as well, but he is avoiding potentially re-infecting his partner by withdrawing before ejaculation. This suggests that they may be using harm reduction strategies.

A behavior whose frequency was of some concern was reported by both HIV-negative and HIV-positive escorts: unprotected oral insertive sex with ejaculation. This behavior has been identified as the least risky method for HIV transmission and infection and many STIs (Halkitis and Parsons, 2000). The higher frequency of this behavior with clients at their request may indicate that the MSW views the behavior as carrying no risk to himself. However, there is no way to ascertain that from this study because it did not measure knowledge of HIV risk.

As is the case with any study of self-reported "high risk" behaviors, the responses of the participants may not be true estimates of the sexual behavior that this study attempted to measure and must therefore be viewed with caution. The cross-sectional design and small sample size also limit the ability to draw definitive causal conclusions from this data. The sample consisted of gay and bisexual male escorts who consented to participate in a research project, and may not be representative of the larger population of gay and bisexual men who advertise their sexual services on the Internet.

Finally, this study is also limited by the questions that were not asked. Intentions for sexual risk behaviors were measured globally and not specifically to partner type. It cannot be known what type of partner the participants were thinking about when they answered the questions regarding their intentions for sexual risk behaviors. Furthermore, this study only sought to explore the relationship between intentions and behavior and not the experiences, beliefs or attitudes that led to these intentions. Lastly, participants were not directly asked "Are you a barebacker?"

In summary, these findings provide an initial understanding regarding the role of intentions for sexual risk behaviors in an understudied group of MSWs: Internet-based male escorts. Based on this study's results, it appears that intervention efforts aiming at having an impact on sexual risk behaviors of gay and bisexual male escorts that should address issues around intentions for engaging in sexual risk behaviors and the reasons behind those intentions, regardless of partner type. Further research studies are needed to ascertain the types of behavioral interventions that would be suitable to these men.

Due to the stigma surrounding sex work, it is unclear if traditional programs such as workshops at gay and lesbian community centers would be well received. MSWs may not be interested in traditional programs typically offered to gay and bisexual men (e.g., small groups, individual counseling, programs focused on condom use) in which one is publicly identified by ones attendance. Instead, new behavioral intervention approaches, perhaps utilizing the Internet, may be required to engage the attention of these particular MSWs since that is the venue in which they are clearly comfortable operating. Finally, barebacking is a relatively recent social and psychological phenomenon. Further clinical work and research will be necessary with gay and bisexual men as a whole to understand the contextual, mental health, and psychosocial factors which contribute to barebacking among gay and bisexual men both in and out of the commercial sex industry.

NOTES

1. A unitary definition of barebacking is essential for developing a concrete understanding of the behavior as well as its prevalence in the gay male community. The most recent edition of *The Joy of Gay Sex* (Silverstein and Picano, 2003) has been updated to include an entry on barebacking and defines it simply as "anal sex without a condom" with no intention implied (p. 1).

2. The text of the following MSW accounts have been edited for clarity, not content. Full transcripts are available.

REFERENCES

Agosto, M. (2001, October). Barebacking is back: The controversy of unprotected sex *Genre*, 97:50.

Allen, D. (1980), Young male prostitutes: A psychosocial study. *Archives Sexual Behavior*, 9:399-426.

Bloor, M., McKeganey, N. & Barnard, M. (1990), An ethnographic study of HIV-related risk practices among Glasgow rent boys and their clients: Report of a pilot study. *AIDS Care*, 2:17-24.

Browne, J. & Minichiello, V. (1996), The social and work context of commercial sex between men: A research note. *Australian & New England J. Sociology*, 32:86-92.

Browne, J. & Minichiello, V. (1995), The Social meanings behind male sex work: Implications for sexual interactions. *British J. Sociology*, 46:598-622.

Calhoun, T.C. & Weaver, G. (1996), Rational decision-making among male street prostitutes. *Deviant Behavior*, 17:209-227.

Caukins, S.E. & Coombs, N.R. (1976) The psychodynamics of male prostitution. *American J. Psychotherapy*, 30:441-451.

Chen, S.Y., Gibson, S., Katz, M.H., Klausner, J.D., Dilley, J.W., Schwarcz, S.K. et al. (2002), Continuing increases in sexual risk behavior and sexually transmitted diseases among men who have sex with men: San Francisco, Calif, 1999-2001. *American J. Public Health*, 92:1387-1388.

Coutinho, R.A., van Andel, R.L.M. & Rijsdijk, T.J. (1988), Role of male prostitutes in the spread of sexually transmitted diseases and human immuno-deficiency virus. *Genitourinary Medicine*, 64:207-208.

Estcourt, C.S., Marks, C., Rohrsheim, R., Johnson, A.M., Donovan, B. & Mindel, A. (2000), HIV, sexually transmitted infections, and risk behaviours in male commercial sex workers in Sydney. *Sexually Transmitted Infections*, 76(4):294-298.

Estep, R., Waldorf, D. & Marotta, T. (1992), Sexual behavior of male prostitutes. In: *The Social Context of AIDS*, eds. J. Huber & B.E. Schneider. Newbury Park, CA: Sage, pp. 95-112.

Gallagher, J. (1998), Risky business. *The Advocate*, p. 46, March 17.

Gauthier, D.K. & Forsyth, C.J. (1999), Bareback sex, bug chasers, and the gift of death. *Deviant Behavior*, 20:85-100.

Gendin, S. (1997), Riding bareback: Skin-on-skin sex been there, done that, want more. *POZ*, pp. 64-65, June.

Gendin, S. (1999), They shoot barebackers don't they? *Poz*, p. 50, February.

Halkitis, P.N. & Parsons, J.T. (2000), Oral sex and HIV risk reduction: Perceived risk, behaviors, and strategies among young HIV negative gay men. *J. Psychology & Human Sexuality*, 11:1-24.

Hickson, F., Weatherburn, P., Hows, J. & Davies, P. (1994), Selling safer sex: Male masseurs and escorts in the UK. In: *Foundations for the Future*, ed. P. Aggleton. Taylor and Francis: London, England, pp. 197-209.

Junge, B. (2002), Bareback sex, risk, and eroticism: Anthropological themes (re-)surfacing in the post-AIDS era. In: *Out in Theory: The Emergence of Lesbian and Gay Anthropology*, eds. E. Lewin & W. Leap. Chicago: University of Illinois Press, pp. 186-221.

Lumby, M.E. (1978), Men who advertise for sex. *Homosexuality*, 4:63-72.

Mansergh, G., Marks, G., Colfax, G., Guzman, R.J., Rader, M. & Buchbinder, S. (2002), Barebacking in a diverse sample of men who have sex with men. *AIDS*, 16:653-659.

Minichiello, V., Marino, R. & Browne, J. (2001), Knowledge, risk perceptions and condom usage in male sex workers from three Australian cities. *AIDS Care*, 13:387-402.

Minichiello, V., Marino, R., Browne, J., Jamieson, M., Peterson, K., Reuter, B. & Robinson, K. (2000), Commercial sex between men: A Prospective diary-based study. *J. Sex Research*, 37:151-160.

Morse, E.V., Simon, P.M., Osofsky, H.J., Balson, P.M. & Gaumer, H.R. (1991), The male street prostitute: A vector for transmission of HIV infection into the heterosexual world. *Social Science & Medicine*, 32:535-539.

Ocamb, K. (1999), Beyond barebacking: The complacency crisis. *Genre*, p. 47, June.

Overs, C. (1991), To work or not to work? Questions facing HIV-positive sex workers. *National AIDS Bulletin*, 5:21.

Parsons, J.T., Bimbi, D.S. & Halkitis, P.N. (2001), Sexual compulsivity among gay/bisexual male escorts who advertise on the internet. *J. Sexual Addiction & Compulsivity*, 8:113-123.

Perkins, R., Prestage, G., Lovejoy, F. & Sharp, R. (1993) Cracking it in the age of AIDS: Female and male prostitutes in the New South Wales commercial sex industry and their responses to HIV prevention. *National AIDS Bulletin*, 7:42-46.

Pleak, R.R. & Meyer-Bahlburg, H.F. (1990), Sexual behavior and AIDS knowledge of young male prostitutes in Manhattan. *J. Sex Research*, 27:557-587.

Rotello, G. (1997), *Sexual Ecology: AIDS and the Destiny of Gay Men*. New York: Dutton.

Salamon, E. (1989), The homosexual escort agency: Deviance disavowal. *British J. Sociology*, 40:2-21.

Savage, D. (1999). Bucking the condomocracy. *Out Magazine*, p. 34, July.

Scarce, M. (1999), A ride on the wild side. *Poz*, p. 52, February.

Silverstein, C. & Picano, F. (2003), *The Joy of Gay Sex, 3rd Edition*. New York: Harper Collins.

Signorile, M. (1998), Sex Panic! and paranoia. *Out Magazine*, pp. 57-61, April.

Suarez, T. & Miller, J. (2001), Negotiating risks in context: A perspective on unprotected anal intercourse and barebacking among men who have sex with men–Where do we go from here? *Archives Sexual Behavior*, 30:287-300.

Warner, M. (1997), Shocked therapy: Finger pointing and shame throwing won't solve the problem of bareback sex. *Poz*, 48, September.

Weisberg, D.K. (1985), *Children of the Night*. Lexington, MA: Lexington Books.

West, D.J. & de Villiers, B. (1993), *Male Prostitution*. Harrington Park Press: New York.

Woltiski, R.J., Valdiserri, R.O., Denning, P.H. & Levine, W.C. (2001), Are we headed for a resurgence in the HIV epidemic among men who have sex with men? *American J. Public Health*, 91:883-888.

Yep, G.A., Lovaas, K.E. & Pagonis, A.V. (2002), The case of "riding bareback": Sexual practices and paradoxes of identity in the era of AIDS. *J. Homosexuality*, 42:1-14.

Ziersch, A., Gaffney, J. & Tomlinson, D.R. (2000), STI prevention and the male sex industry in London: Evaluating a pilot peer education program. *Sexually Transmitted Infections*, 76:447-453.

Attitudes Toward Unprotected
Anal Intercourse:
Assessing HIV-Negative Gay
or Bisexual Men

Ariel Shidlo, PhD
Huso Yi, PhD
Boaz Dalit, PsyD

SUMMARY. HIV prevention programs and clinicians have a need to identify clients' attitudes toward unprotected anal intercourse (UAI). This study reports on the development of the Unprotected Anal Intercourse Attitudes Inventory (UAI-AI), a multi-factorial measure designed to assess gay and bisexual men who are HIV-negative or

---

Ariel Shidlo and Huso Yi are affiliated with TalkSafe, New York City.

Boaz Dalit is in Independent Practice in New York City.

Address correspondence to: Ariel Shidlo, PhD, 420 West 24th Street, Suite 1B, New York, NY 10011 (E-mail: ashidlo@aol.com).

The authors express gratitude to Jim Jasper for his invaluable editorial advice. Henry Koegel assisted in the collection of these data and introduced the Beck Depression Inventory into the assessment battery used on intake at TalkSafe.

TalkSafe is supported by the Centers for Disease Control and Prevention (CDC) grant funding, given through the New York City Department of Health to the Medical and Health Research Association of New York City, Inc. The contents of this study are solely the responsibility of TalkSafe and do not necessarily represent the official views of the funders.

[Haworth co-indexing entry note]: "Attitudes Toward Unprotected Anal Intercourse: Assessing HIV-Negative Gay or Bisexual Men." Shidlo, Ariel, Huso Yi, and Boaz Dalit. Co-published simultaneously in *Journal of Gay & Lesbian Psychotherapy* (The Haworth Medical Press, an imprint of The Haworth Press, Inc.) Vol. 9, No. 3/4, 2005, pp. 107-128; and: *Barebacking: Psychosocial and Public Health Approaches* (ed: Perry N. Halkitis, Leo Wilton, and Jack Drescher) The Haworth Medical Press, an imprint of The Haworth Press, Inc., 2005, pp. 107-128. Single or multiple copies of this article are available for a fee from The Haworth Document Delivery Service [1-800-HAWORTH, 9:00 a.m. - 5:00 p.m. (EST). E-mail address: docdelivery@haworthpress.com].

untested. This self-report measure may be useful in helping both counselors and clients discuss the complex psychosocial issues that can be associated with UAI and safer sex. Factors identified include Anger/Self-Destructiveness/Fatalism, Pleasure Seeking/Risk-Taking/Escapism, Intimacy Needs/Rational Choice Making, Erroneous Perception of Risk, and Condom Related Erectile Dysfunction. Based on their work with hundreds of clients at TalkSafe, a NYC prevention program for HIV-negative gay and bisexual men, the authors suggest clinical guidelines for counseling these populations. *[Article copies available for a fee from The Haworth Document Delivery Service: 1-800-HAWORTH. E-mail address: <docdelivery@haworthpress.com> Website: <http://www.HaworthPress.com>* © *2005 by The Haworth Press, Inc. All rights reserved.]*

KEYWORDS. AIDS, anal intercourse, barebacking, gay and bisexual men, high-risk sexual behavior, HIV-negative MSM, homosexuality, safer sex, STI, Unprotected Anal Intercourse Attitudes Inventory

The seroconversion rate for HIV among gay and bisexual men in the United States (U.S.) has continued to grow over the past several years (CDC, 2003; Chen et al., 2002; Halkitis, Parsons and Wilton, 2003; Kellogg et al., 2001). Wolitski et al. (2001) state that "there are indications that we may be headed for a resurgence of HIV infections among MSM" (p. 883). These indicators include increases in sexually transmitted infections (STIs) and high levels of unprotected anal intercourse (UAI) with partners of unknown or different HIV serostatus than oneself (Halkitis et al., 2004; Turner et al., 2003). In response to the growing realization that information-based prevention campaigns are not sufficient, the first author of this study founded TalkSafe in 1995. TalkSafe is a secondary prevention program for HIV-negative gay and bisexual men in New York City that provides intensive psychological counseling. The program's guiding principle is that remaining HIV-negative is best accomplished by promoting the establishment of an HIV-negative identity. Counseling helps clients integrate an HIV-negative identity with their identities as gay and bisexual men through tailored interventions consisting of individual, couple, and group counseling. Every client is assessed before treatment to determine the unique factors that place them at risk for HIV. These factors include attitudes toward being HIV-negative, self-esteem, internalized homophobia, intimacy issues, relationship skills, assertiveness, substance abuse, mental disorders, and attitudes toward UAI (Odets, 1995; Shidlo, 1997).

To facilitate assessment of attitudes toward UAI, Shidlo and Dalit (1996) developed a 41-item self-report measure, the Unprotected Anal Intercourse Attitudes Inventory (UAI-AI). The UAI-AI was designed to capture the heterogeneity of justifications for UAI among HIV-negative gay and bisexual men. Based on clinical work, 12 theoretical factors for the measure were identified:

1. *Erroneous perception of non-riskiness of partner or sexual behavior* assesses how individuals evaluate risk based on the looks, age, or behavior of their partner (i.e., not offering to use a condom);
2. *Self-destructive impulses* and
3. *Other-destructive impulses* refer to when these impulses lead individuals to view HIV infection as a means of punishing oneself or others;
4. *AIDS fatigue* or weariness occurs when competing needs for vigilance in sexual contact and the desire for pleasure and escape in sex;
5. *Need for intimacy* relates to how condoms are experienced as barriers and the desire to abandon normal boundaries and merge with another person;
6. *Rational risk-taking* occurs when an HIV-negative individual determines accurately that his sexual partner does not pose a risk for HIV infection;
7. *Diminished self-control* refers to when normal abilities to protect oneself against the danger of HIV infection are affected by substances or especially intense states of sexual arousal;
8. *Sense of invulnerability* develops out of repeated UAI and subsequent HIV-negative test results;
9. *Assertiveness failure* occurs when one's sexual partner insists on UAI or appears disinterested in using condoms;
10. *Sense of fatalism* occurs due to a loss of peers to AIDS or to a lack of faith in prevention messages that may be seen as inconclusive (transmission of HIV through oral sex, for instance);
11. *Condom-related erectile dysfunction* affects the insertive partner during anal intercourse. Some gay and bisexual men find it impossible to sustain an erection when they attempt to use a condom and consequently abandon condom use due to frustration and embarrassment; and
12. Other condom-related attitudes, such as perception of partner's interest in using condoms.

In order to begin the process of evaluating the construct validity of the UAI-AI, an exploratory factor analysis was conducted. The primary goal was to determine whether the factor structure in this sample corresponded to the theoretical subscales predicted. Subsequently, the internal consistency and construct validity of the empirically derived subscales generated from the factor analysis were examined. Because the social phenomenon of "barebacking" appeared after the initial version of the UAI-AI was developed, these data do not reflect attitudes toward barebacking. Nonetheless, we share our thoughts on the implications of barebacking on clinical work and research, and also present clinical guidelines for use with HIV-negative MSM derived from our work in counseling these individuals.

METHOD

Participants

Participants were clients of TalkSafe, a secondary prevention program in NYC that provides peer counseling to HIV-negative and untested gay and bisexual men. Clients who reported having engaged in UAI completed the UAI-AI. Unfortunately, data is unavailable on the frequency of UAI or whether ejaculation occurred. An examination of the 207 available UAI-AI protocols revealed that participants who completed 13 or less of the total 41 items appeared to have done so in a haphazard way (i.e., several groups of three items all endorsed exactly the same on the Likert scale). Therefore, eight protocols were excluded from the analyses resulting in a final sample of 199. Mean substitution was used for missing values. One-hundred-and-ninety (96%) participants reported having tested HIV-negative and 7 (4%) were untested. With regard to sexual orientation, 181 (91%) self-identified as gay, 4 (2%) as homosexual, and 11 (6%) as bisexual. The ethnic background of participants included 115 (58%) White, 25 (13%) African American, 38 (19%) Latino/Hispanic, 4 (2%) Asian and Pacific Islander, 2 (1%) Native American, and 9 (5%) multi- or other ethnicities. The average age of the participants was 35 (SD = 8.4) with a range of 18 to 66. In terms of education level, 6 (3%) completed high school, 74 (37%) completed 1-4 years of college, and 40 (20%) completed some graduate studies. Relationship status of the participants included 139 (70%) single men and 54 (27%) in a primary relationship; of those in a relationship, 17 (9%) reported cohabiting. Forty (20%) participants had one sexual partner, 131 (66%) reported multiple partners, and 25 (13%) were celibate. With regard to "outness" about sexual orientation, 181 (91%) were out to gay or bisexual friends, 149 (75%) to heterosexual friends, 162 (81%) to family, 113 (57%) to co-workers. Only one subject was not out to anyone. Percentages do not add up to 100 because of missing data.

Procedure and Measures

All clients who presented for counseling at TalkSafe were interviewed by a clinician as a part of an intake procedure that involved the completion of a battery of self-report measures. These measures included an assessment of sexual risk behavior, sexual orientation, and drug use.[1] Depression was assessed using the Beck Depression Inventory (BDI; Beck, 1972). Internalized homophobia was measured by the Multi-Axial Gay Attitudes Inventory-Men's Short Version (MAGAI-MSV), a 20-item self-report instrument using a 4-point Likert scale. This measure has shown adequate internal consistency (alpha = .87) and preliminary construct validity (Shidlo and Hollander, 1998).

Attitudes toward UAI were assessed using a newly created self-administered instrument, the Unprotected Anal Intercourse Attitudes Inventory (UAI-AI). Based on our clinical work, 12 theoretical factors and developed 41 corresponding items were identified (see Table 1). Participants were asked to "Think back to the last time that you had anal intercourse without a condom, and try to be as honest as you can in marking which statements describe why you didn't use a condom." A 4-point Likert scale was used: 4 (*Strongly Agree*), 3 (*Mainly Agree*), 2 (*Mainly Disagree*), and 1 (*Strongly Disagree*).

RESULTS

Table 1 lists the UAI-AI items. An exploratory factor analysis (PCA) was used to determine how many interpretable factors explained the variance in the items above. Subsequently, these empirically generated factors were compared with the initial theoretical factors. Five factors were retained based on an examination of Catelli's (1966) scree test, Kaiser's eigenvalue rule (DeVellis, 1991), and comprehensibility. The lowest eigenvalue of the five factors retained was 1.91. The cumulative percentage of the variance explained by the five *unrotated* factors was 45.20. Varimax was used to rotate the factors to yield an interpretable solution. After rotation, the lowest eigenvalue was 2.34. The following

TABLE 1. UAI-AI Theoretical Factors

Theoretical factor (TF) and items	MEAN	SD
TF1–Erroneous Perception of Risk		
I assumed he was HIV-negative too	2.69	1.25
He seemed too young to be HIV-positive	1.47	.91
We were in love and assumed we were...	1.84	1.20
He told me he was HIV-negative	2.27	1.31
He seemed too healthy to be infected	1.92	1.05
TF2–Condom Related Erectile Dysfunction		
The condom didn't fit right	1.20	.62
I can't get hard when I think about a condom	1.64	.97
I can't stay hard when I put a condom on	1.79	1.03
TF3–Intimacy Need		
We wanted to feel each other without a condom...	2.65	1.24
I just wanted to feel what it was like without...	2.33	1.26
I wanted to feel him coming inside me	1.69	1.13
I wanted to be closer to my partner who is...	1.19	.62
We wanted to feel closer to each other	2.15	1.18
TF4–Rational Risk Taking		
My boyfriend and I are both HIV-negative...	1.84	1.25
I felt like I was making a choice not to use...	2.17	1.18
TF5–Self-Destructive Impulses/Negative Affect		
I was feeling depressed and self-destructive	1.83	1.10
I just didn't care about myself that much	1.82	1.08
I wanted to hurt myself	1.40	.77
I was feeling guilty about being HIV-negative	1.24	.62
I was high and just didn't care	1.50	.91
TF6–Other-Destructive Impulses		
I was feeling angry at everybody	1.49	.89
I wanted to hurt my partner	1.17	.56
I probably am HIV-positive, so why shouldn't others...	1.11	.46
I just didn't care about my partner that much	1.36	.74

Theoretical factor (TF) and items	MEAN	SD
TF7–AIDS Fatigue		
I wanted to forget about AIDS	1.94	1.14
I was too happy to deal with condoms and AIDS	1.74	1.02
TF8–Diminished Self-Control		
I was very horny that night and found it hard to control...	2.64	1.18
The guy was really hot	2.36	1.17
I was too loaded or drunk	1.43	.88
TF9–Sense of Invulnerability		
I've gotten away with it before	2.17	1.14
I wanted to see if I could get away with it and not get...	1.49	.84
I didn't think it would be risky if we didn't come inside...	2.07	1.15
I was the top, so I didn't feel that it was risky to me	2.08	1.11
TF10–Assertiveness Failure		
He insisted that we fuck without condoms and I just...	1.60	.97
I felt uncomfortable talking about condoms	1.61	.97
I didn't want him to think that I am HIV-positive	1.29	.69
TF11–Fatalism (Lack of Faith in Prevention)		
I don't think safer sex will protect me anyway	1.25	.63
AIDS is going to get me no matter what	1.33	.67
TF12–Other Condom-Related Items		
I didn't remember to use a condom	1.35	.73
I didn't have a condom	1.67	1.06
The other guy didn't seem to care about condoms	2.33	1.20

Note. The range on each item is 1 to 4, with 1 = "Strongly Disagree" and 4 = "Strongly Agree."

are the item loadings for each factor, with the percentage of the variance of each factor after the factor description (see Table 2).

Five items showed correlations (above .38) with multiple factors and were dropped because this suggests that they were not uni-dimensional and need to be re-written: (1) "I was feeling depressed and self-destructive"; (2) "I just didn't care about myself that much" (factors 1 and 2); (3) "I just wanted to see what it was like without the condom" (factors 2 and 3); (4) "I was too happy to deal with condoms and AIDS" (factors 2 and 4); and (5) "I was too loaded or drunk" (factors 1 and 4).

TABLE 2. Factor Loadings for UAI-AI

	Factor Loading	Percentage of Variance
Factor 1: Anger/Self-Destructiveness/Fatalism		12.69%
I wanted to hurt myself	.76	
I wanted to hurt my partner	.73	
I probably am HIV-positive so why shouldn't...	.69	
I was feeling angry at everybody	.68	
I don't think safer sex will protect me anyway	.57	
I just didn't care about my partner that much	.57	
AIDS is going to get me no matter what	.53	
I was feeling guilty about being HIV-negative	.46	
I was high and just didn't care	.43	
Factor 2: Pleasure Seeking/Risk-Taking/Escapism		10.48%
I was very horny that night and found it hard...	.69	
I've gotten away with it before	.68	
The guy was really hot	.63	
The other guy didn't seem to care about...	.60	
I wanted to forget about AIDS	.53	
I wanted to see if I could get away with it...	.41	
Factor 3: Intimacy Needs/Rational Choice Making		8.30%
We wanted to feel each other without a...	.72	
We wanted to feel closer to each other	.71	
My boyfriend and I are both negative...	.65	
I wanted to feel him coming inside me	.61	
We were in love and assumed we were both...	.57	
He told me was HIV-negative	.55	
I felt like I was making a choice not to use...	.48	
Factor 4: Erroneous Perception of Risk		8.03%
He seemed too healthy to be infected	.69	
He seemed too young to be HIV-positive	.65	
I assumed he was HIV-negative too	.43	
I didn't think it would be risky if we didn't...	.31	
Factor 5: Condom-Related Erectile Dysfunction		5.71%
I can't stay hard when I put a condom on	.86	
I can't get hard when I put a condom on	.85	
The condom didn't fit right	.41	

Three items were dropped because, although they showed satisfactory correlations with only one factor, they made the factor difficult to interpret: (1) "I didn't want him to think that I was HIV-positive"; (2) "I didn't have a condom"; and (3) "I didn't remember to use a condom."

Finally, four items were excluded because of low correlations (below .4) with any factor and because they hindered comprehensibility of the solution: (1) "I wanted to be closer to my partner who is HIV-positive"; (2) "He insisted that we fuck without condoms and I just couldn't say no"; (3) "I was the top so I didn't feel that it was risky to me; and (4) I felt uncomfortable talking about condoms." Since the current factor solution is only an exploratory one, it is possible that when replicated with a larger sample, these items might prove useful in another factor solution. Therefore, these items will be retained in the scale when re-administered in the future.

Because factor five contains only three variables (see Table 2), it should be interpreted with great caution as the likelihood for unreliability is high (Tabachnick and Fidell, 1983). It has been tentatively retained because the dimension it represents, condom-related erectile dysfunction, is important and merits creating additional items to test using factor analytic methods with a new sample.

Since Varimax rotation makes an assumption of the orthogonality of factors, an important question is to what extent these factors actually correlate with each other. Following the recommendation of Tabachnick and Fidell (1983), the component score correlation matrix generated by an oblique rotation (Oblimin) was examined; the five factors were found to have correlations below .30. This suggests that the factors can be interpreted as orthogonal and a Varimax rotation is appropriate.

Subsequently, reliability analysis was done to check for the internal consistency of each subscale (see Table 3). Using DeVellis's (1991) guidelines for evaluating alpha levels, the pattern of coefficients suggest that factor 1 is in the "very good range," factors 2, 3, and 5 in the "acceptable" range, and factor 4 has "unacceptably low" internal consistency. For factor 4, when the item "I assumed he was HIV-negative too" is dropped, the standardized alpha shows a slight improvement (.63) but still in the undesirable range.

Construct Validity

To assess the construct validity of the UAI-AI, we conducted several analyses of the relationship of its subscales with other variables that are

TABLE 3. Internal Consistency of the Five PCA Factors

Factor	Adjusted Alpha	Scale Mean	SD	No. of Items
1: Anger/self-destructiveness/fatalism	.83	11.71	3.98	9
2: Pleasure seeking/risk-taking/escapism	.78	12.81	4.62	6
3: Intimacy needs/rational choice making	.76	14.57	5.47	7
4: Erroneous perception of risk	.59	8.11	2.90	4
5: Condom-related erectile dysfunction	.73	4.63	2.19	3

conceptually related. Scores on the *Pleasure seeking/risk-taking/escapism* subscale were predicted to be significantly higher among those who reported drug use. A proxy variable was created to group all participants who reported using any of the following: cannabis, cocaine IN, cocaine IV, heroin IN, heroin IV, crack, ecstasy, LSD, K, or crystal methamphetamine. Forty participants reported using at least one of the above substances. An independent samples t-test did not show a significant difference between *Pleasure seeking/risk-taking/escapism* levels in the drug using group (M = 12.72, SD = 4.31) and the non-drug using group (M = 12.93, SD = 4.79). In fact, there was a puzzling trend of a higher, but non-significant escapism mean scores among the group that did *not* report using drugs. This negative result may be due to the fact that we did not have a robust indicator of substance abuse but rather only of substance use. Thus, the data on substance use did not differentiate between occasional use of substances and significant abuse.

It was expected that participants who reported drug use would show higher scores on the subscale *Anger/self-destructiveness/fatalism* as compared to non drug users. The results were consistent with this prediction, but the difference did not achieve significance (drug-users M = 12.32, SD = 4.13 versus non-drug-users M = 11.5, SD = 3.92).

The *Anger/self-destructiveness/fatalism* subscale was predicted to be positively correlated with level of internalized homophobia. This relationship was expected because internalized homophobia has shown a variety of positive correlations with measures of dysfunction and subjective distress (Shidlo, 1994). The results showed a modest significant positive correlation (r = .22, p < .01, n = 135).

Another expected relationship was a positive correlation between the subscale *Anger/self-destructiveness/fatalism* and scores on the Beck

Depression Inventory. This was supported by a small but significant association (r = .26, p < .005, n = 114).

DISCUSSION

The current results suggest that the UAI-AI has preliminary promise as an assessment tool in clinical and prevention settings with HIV-negative or untested gay and bisexual men. The five factors based on this factor analytic solution are consistent with our theoretical predictions (see Table 4): (1) Anger/self-destructiveness/fatalism, (2) Pleasure seeking/risk-taking/escapism, (3) Intimacy needs/rational choice making, (4) Erroneous perception of risk, and (5) Condom-related erectile dysfunction. These results support our model of attitudes toward UAI as one that is multi-dimensional.

Why is it important to emphasize (what may be intuitively obvious) that UAI is engaged in for many different reasons rather than a single psychological factor? Because subgroups of individuals may engage in UAI for dissimilar motivations, it is likely that prevention messages and interventions that are diffuse and too generalized may not be very effective. When planning interventions and prevention messages for HIV-negative MSM, we would recommend the development of a series of modules and message types that address each of the UAI factors that we or other researchers have identified as strongly associated with risk behavior.

How did the factors obtained in this study compare with those identified in previous research? In a pioneering publication in this area, Gold et al. (1991) identified the following four factors: (1) inferring whether the partner is likely to be infected with HIV from personal characteristics; (2) bargaining or special pleading for protection from HIV based on past efforts at safer sex; (3) fear of making a negative impression on a partner; and (4) perceiving oneself as immune or protected from HIV infection. Three of these factors are consistent with factors we obtained through PCA: Pleasure seeking/risk-taking/escapism, Erroneous perception of risk, and Pleasure seeking/risk-taking/escapism (see Table 4).

Dilley et al. (2002) created a 102-item scale based on the work of Gold et al. (1991) and reported on several theoretically-derived subscales that demonstrated an alpha coefficient of at least .70: condoms reduce sexual pleasure; fatalism; loss of control; inferring that the partner is not likely to be HIV-infected based on looks, speech, or behavior; low

TABLE 4. Comparison of Theoretical and PCA Factors in This Study to Results of Other Researchers

Theoretical Factors	PCA Factors	Comparable Factors Found by Other Researchers
Erroneous perception of risk	Erroneous perception of risk	Dilley et al. (2002)[T] Gold et al. (1991)[FA] Suarez & Miller (2001)[T]
Condom-related erectile dysfunction	Condom-related erectile dysfunction	
Intimacy need	Intimacy needs and rational choice making	Dilley et al. (2002)[T]
Rational risk taking	Intimacy needs and rational choice making	Dilley et al. (2002)[T] Suarez and Miller (2001)[T]
Self-destructive impulses	Anger, self-destructiveness, and negative affect	Dilley et al. (2002)[T]
Other-destructive impulses	Anger, self-destructiveness, and fatalism	
AIDS fatigue	Pleasure seeking, risk-taking, and escapism	Dilley et al. (2002)[T]
Diminished self-control		Dilley et al. (2002)[T]
Sense of invulnerability	Pleasure seeking, risk-taking, and escapism	Gold et al. (1991)[FA]
Assertiveness failure		Gold et al. (1991)[FA]
Fatalism (lack of faith in prevention)	Anger, self-destructiveness, and fatalism	Dilley et al. (2002)[T] Kalichman et al. (1997)[ANC]
Other condom-related items		

Note. FA = Factor Analysis ; T = Theoretical Factor; ANC = Ancova.

self-esteem; non-prescribed safer sex methods or beliefs; inferring that the partner is not infected based on information; exhaustion at maintaining safer sex; intimacy and emotional needs for unprotected sex; new HIV treatments; and favorable attitude toward being HIV infected. Table 3 shows the matching points of our PCA-derived factors with Dilley and his colleagues' theoretical factors. Dilley et al. reported that they did not find a robust factor analysis solution for these items. Although many reasons can account for this, this may be due to the low ratio of subject number to number of scale items in their study (a ratio of approximately 2.5 participants per item).

Shifting back to evaluating our new instrument, the UAI-AI, one limitation of this study is that since the factor analysis was done on one sample, the results may be unstable or artifacts of this unique sample. As always, when developing a new measure, replication with other clinical and non-clinical samples is essential to evaluate the stability of the factor solution and construct validity.

Nonetheless, we found additional preliminary evidence of construct validity, whereby the UAI-AI subscale of *Anger/self-destructiveness/ fatalism* was positively correlated with internalized homophobia and level of depression. The relationship between depression and sexual behavior is beyond the scope of this paper and needs to be further studied (cf. Bancroft et al., 2003). With regards to drug use, scores on the subscales *Anger/self-destructiveness/fatalism* and *Pleasure seeking/ risk-taking/escapism* did not differentiate between participants who *used* substances and those who did not. However, an important limitation of our data is that we cannot differentiate between participants who used substances and those who abused them. Therefore, these subscales need to be further tested by comparing participants who *abuse* substances with those who do not.

One final limitation is that our work on the UAI-AI started in the mid 1990s before the use of the term barebacking was widespread. Therefore, our instrument did not include an assessment of this phenomenon. In 2004, we intend to update the UAI-AI by adding items that tap this dimension. We therefore follow with our preliminary thoughts on the conceptual challenges of understanding and assessing barebacking.

SOME THOUGHTS ON BAREBACKING

Barebacking has been defined as *intentional* unprotected anal intercourse (UAI) in order to differentiate it from that UAI which reflects a *relapse* from safer sex norms. We believe that there is a further distinction that is important: barebacking as a *behavior* versus barebacker as an *identity* (Halkitis, Parsons and Wilton, 2003; Halkitis et al., 2005). To illustrate the difference between barebacking behavior and a barebacker identity, consider that some individuals may intend to engage in UAI and yet not consider the behavior as "barebacking" or themselves to be "barebackers." An HIV-negative man may have intentional UAI with an HIV-negative partner whom he trusts and reject the barebacking label because it is based on a rational assessment of low or no risk. Conversely, an HIV-positive man may intentionally have UAI with a partner who is HIV-negative or of unknown status because he feels angry at the world, and subsequently feels guilt and shame about his behavior. This HIV-positive individual would not view himself as a barebacker but as someone who engaged in UAI during a difficult emotional state. From a public health perspective, this individual may be viewed as someone who has relapsed even though his behavior was intentional. This sub-group of individuals who have engaged in intentional UAI experiences the behavior as ego-dystonic, or alien to their sense of self, and does not identify as barebackers. In contrast, a barebacker assumes an identity as someone who practices intentional UAI and experiences it as ego-syntonic, or consistent with his sense of self: "I have bareback sex because this is who I am."

To provide a sense of the ethos of individuals who identify as barebackers, a brief text analysis of the words of the founders of a popular barebacking website is presented here (barebackcity.com, retrieved on August 3, 2003): "We are here for those who want to live this lifestyle, and don't feel that they fit into the 'safe-sex world.'" These words express a need to belong to a community in which their views on unprotected intercourse are unchallenged. One distinguishing feature of many barebackers is the unapologetic nature of their views on unprotected sex. This website's introduction reads: "No excuses! No justifications!" The website dismisses concerns about AID, saying: "What about it? It will still exist if we have this site up or not." It speaks to the reader's sense of autonomy and choice: "It's up to you (remember, you are an adult, aren't you) to decide how you want to run your life, who you want to fuck, whom you infect, and what you even believe." It explicitly rejects safer sex as not having a place in their community and threatens users with expulsion if they mention safer sex in their online personal ads: "If your ad indicates 'safe sex only' . . . If caught, your listing will be deleted, your account will be deleted, AND you will be banned from this site." In sum, we believe that although intentionality is a necessary component in conceptualizing barebacking, it is not sufficient. An identity as a barebacker and lack of remorse or distress about intentional UAI are the additional necessary components.

How does the concept of *intentionality* intersect with the theoretical factors used to develop the UAI-AI? Based on the theoretical factors identified in developing the UAI-AI, only *Rational risk-taking* appears, by definition, to be associated with intentionality. In contrast, three factors appear to be always associated with *non-intentional behavior*: (1) Erroneous perception of non-riskiness of partner or sexual behavior, (2) Diminished self-control, and (3) Assertiveness failure. As opposed to the above factors, six factors can be associated with *either intentional or non-intentional behavior*: (1) self-destructive impulses and other-destructive impulses, (2) AIDS fatigue, (3) need for intimacy, (4) a sense of invulnerability, (5) a sense of fatalism, and (6) condom-related erectile dysfunction. In our next study, we intend to assess respondents' level of identification as barebackers and determine how this dimension relates to the UAI-AI factors we have conceptualized thus far. We also plan a closer study of the concept of intentionality in UAI.

CLINICAL RECOMMENDATIONS

Although the UAI-AI is in the piloting stages of establishing construct validity, clinicians who work with HIV-negative or untested gay and bisexual men may find it helpful. As scoring is not essential to make it useful clinically, the instrument can be easily administered and help sensitize both the client and clinician to critical attitudes toward UAI. A joint in-session review of responses may be helpful in starting a conversation about these issues and, when needed, focusing the therapy on the determinants of risky sex. Most importantly, the administration of the UAI-AI may also communicate to clients that the therapist is open to discussing a topic that is frequently associated with secretiveness and shame. At TalkSafe, many of our HIV-negative and untested gay and bisexual clients reported that they had not discussed their feelings about being HIV-negative in previous courses of psychotherapy *because their therapist had not raised the issue*. Therefore, we conclude by offering clinical guidelines for clinicians who are working with these populations. These guidelines are of course not intended as a "cookbook" on psychotherapy but may serve as useful issues to integrate, as needed, into treatment:

1. *Examine your clients' attitudes regarding their HIV-negative serostatus.* Gay men who are HIV-negative may experience a multitude of conflicting feelings about their serostatus. Encourage your client to articulate both negative and positive feelings about being seronegative and to tolerate the confusion of contradictory sentiments. The following dimensions bear assessment: (a) guilt, shame, and secrecy about being seronegative; (b) precariousness about HIV-negative serostatus; and (c) trivializing the struggle to remain HIV-negative, when compared to the concerns of others who are HIV-positive.

2. *Promote the integration of an HIV-negative identity.* HIV-negative gay men need help to develop an identity that integrates being uninfected into other aspects of their lives. They need to be given permission to feel that being HIV-negative is something that they can feel good about and tell others. An adaptive identity integration of an HIV seronegative status can only be accomplished after exploring emotional states such as depression, anxiety, and loneliness. Facilitate the process of grieving the intrusiveness of AIDS on love, dating, relationships, sex, and sense of self.

3. *Encourage clients to explore the meanings of barebacking and assess whether they view it as syntonic or dystonic with their identity.* Clients who perceive themselves as being "conformists" in their values (e.g., holding a professional job, being law abiding, being disciplined in their careers, treating others with kindness) may experience barebacking as an exciting form of social rebellion. Help these HIV-negative clients search for less self-destructive ways of expressing their vitality.

4. *Identify errors in communication.* Many HIV-negative gay men interpret the willingness of a sexual partner to have unprotected anal intercourse with them as evidence that their partner is also seronegative (Gold, 1995). The assumption is that their sexual partner is *the same as them*–seronegative. Your clients need to be educated that their seropositive partners may make an assumption of *sameness of serostatus* and think: "You're willing to have unprotected anal intercourse? This must mean *you are the same as me*; we are both HIV-positive so it's OK to do it without a condom." Help your client to feel comfortable discussing serostatus issues with sexual partners.

5. *Help your clients articulate the meanings of specific sexual behavior.* Your clients may appear comfortable talking about sex but have difficulty exploring the meanings that concrete sexual acts

hold for them. Each gay man may have a unique constellation of meanings attached to sex and AIDS. Help your clients articulate aloud what anal intercourse with and without a condom means to them, what oral sex with and without a condom means to them, what having men ejaculate inside them means to them, what ejaculating inside another man means to them, what kissing another man means to them, and what being sexually desired by another man means to them. Ask what it means to them to have sex with an HIV-negative partner, HIV-positive partner, and a partner of unknown serostatus (Elovich, 1995).

6. *Discuss oral sex transmission data and prevention guidelines and address the psychological impact resulting from their ambiguity.* Many gay men have considerable anxiety about unprotected oral sex because the evidence about transmission is ambiguous. The *de facto* standard of safer sex among many gay men includes unprotected oral sex. Examine whether anxiety and anger about the ambiguity of the riskiness of oral sex leads your client to engage in UAI ("No one knows what's really safe anyway; I might as well have anal intercourse without a condom").

7. *If appropriate, establish guidelines for negotiated safety.* Clinicians need to acknowledge that many HIV-negative gay men are using their own heuristics to estimate risk and guide their decisions about UAI. For example, monogamous couples where both partners have tested HIV-negative sometimes choose to have UAI. In order to minimize the risks of this decision, they need to be encouraged to think through and talk openly about their choice. The Victorian AIDS Council/Gay Men's Health Centre in Australia (Victorian AIDS Council, 1994) has helpful education for couples considering UAI. They recognize that issues of trust and communication are crucial in decisions to have UAI. Our adaptation of their guidelines is as follows: (a) the couple discusses the importance and meanings of UAI for each of the partners; (b) if they both strongly want to engage in UAI, both partners have an HIV test (preferably together) and commit to be completely honest with each other about the results; (c) the couple continues to use condoms every time they have anal intercourse for six months; (d) the couple has another HIV test together; (e) if both test seronegative, the couple agrees that neither partner will engage in UAI outside the relationship; (f) *the couple commits and promises to tell each other immediately if this agreement is broken*, re-start condoms for anal sex, and go through steps "1" to "5"

again; (g) if both partners have HIV they should consider the effects of reinfection when deciding about UAI with each other; and (h) if one of the partners is HIV seropositive, they should continue to use condoms every time they have anal intercourse.

8. *Help your clients assess the unique factors that might lead them to engage in UAI with a partner of unknown status or a seropositive partner.* Each individual differs on the relative importance of the factors that may be associated with UAI: (a) internalized homonegativity (Shidlo, 1994): negative attitudes toward one's homosexual feelings, behavior, relationships, and identity; (b) shame about sex with other men; (c) hopelessness and indifference about the future and one's personal well-being; fatigue of living in an epidemic without an apparent end: "We'll all get it sooner or later, it's just a question of time"; (d) difficulty in forming a healthy identity as an HIV-negative gay man: experience of shame, secrecy, guilt, isolation, alienation, and lack of visible role models (Odets, 1995); (e) difficulty saying no to an attractive or sexually desirable partner who requests UAI; (f) experience of rejection by other gay men and associated negative mood states (Gold, 1995; Odets, 1995); (g) impact of body image: poor body image may increase vulnerability to risky UAI; (h) risk-seeking trait and sexual adventurism, or the need for exciting or novel sexual situations (Halkitis and Parsons, 2003; Ostrow, DiFranceisco and Kalichman (1997); (i) communication and assertiveness skills: difficulty asking a partner's serostatus, telling a partner one's status, initiating condom use, insisting on condom use; (j) informational fallacies: erroneous beliefs that insertive partners ("tops") can't get infected in UAI, UAI without ejaculation is safe, and UAI limited to insertion of tip of penis is OK; (k) invulnerability: sense of personal immunity sometimes confirmed by repeated HIV seronegative test results in spite of history of risky UAI; (l) untreated depressive disorder; (m) untreated substance and alcohol abuse or dependence (Ostrow et al.,1997); (n) need for intimacy: closeness and feeling of trust provided by UAI takes on paramount significance over longevity and health (Odets, 1995). For some men, exchange of sperm may be strongly valued; (o) perception of masculinity as defined by sexual competency (Halkitis, 2001): HIV-positive men who report perceiving their masculinity as affirmed by sexual activity have been found to be more likely to engage in UAI (Halkitis and Parsons, 2003); a similar process may affect HIV-negative men; (p) negative associations with con-

dom use: some men may view condoms as signifying "promiscuity," lack of trust, betrayal and evidence of unacknowledged seropositivity in partner; (q) condom-associated sexual dysfunction: erectile difficulties in the insertive partner; and (r) inter-ethnic negative attitudes: differential perception of seroprevalence in a particular ethnic group; sadistic or masochistic impulses toward the partner of a different ethnicity.

9. *Conceptualize how characterological and developmental issues may be exacerbated by AIDS-related issues.* Help clients identify which aspects of their psychological distress or maladaptive behavior are in direct response to the stresses of the AIDS epidemic versus those aspects that are a re-activation of earlier wounds and vulnerabilities. Assess whether earlier developmental issues related to internalized homophobia and gay identity formation need to be revisited. For some clients, AIDS may serve as a repository of toxic material. Ball (1995) reports having seen clients whose previous therapists interpreted anxiety, panic, and depression as solely characterological in origin, failing to contextualize them as normal reactions to the ongoing traumatization of the AIDS epidemic.

10. *Actively support your clients when they report dating, falling in love, being in relationships, and having sex.* Gay men need to hear that loving other men is a good thing and that sex with other men is a healthy and desirable thing. In the context of the "AIDSification of gay identity" and "homosexualization of AIDS" (Odets, 1995), it is an essential function for the provider to act as a counterforce that helps the client celebrate being gay or bisexual. Challenge the tendency of clients to pathologize their relationships and sexual behavior. Help them examine what they actually mean when they report that they are "addicted" to sex. Is this an accurate description of dyscontrol and compulsion, or an AIDS-phobic and gay-phobic misinterpretation of high levels of sexual desire?

11. *Assess clients' needs for individual, couple, and group modalities.* Clients early in the process of examining issues about being seronegative may require individual intervention. Offer couple counseling for seronegative and mixed serostatus couples. Stating the obvious, not all HIV-negative gay men are appropriate for a group intervention. Screening for membership in group should be conducted according to established principles (Yalom, 1995).

12. *Design primary prevention programs and counseling materials that explicitly recognize HIV-negative gay men and HIV-positive*

gay men and target each population distinctly (Odets,1995). Avoid obfuscating the differences between the concerns and feelings of HIV negative and -positive gay men. HIV-negative men need to be helped to value self-preservation in addition to supporting their HIV-positive peers. HIV-positive men need to be helped to value avoiding re-infection with HIV or exposure to other STIs in addition to maintaining the health of their HIV-negative peers.

NOTE

1. Please contact the authors for more information on our clinical assessment battery.

REFERENCES

Ball, S. (1995), Positively negative. *In the Family*, 1:22-25, October 14-17.

Bancroft, J., Janssen, E., Strong, D. & Vukadinovic, Z. (2003), The relation between mood and sexuality in gay men. *Archives Sexual Behavior*, 32:231-242.

Beck, A.T. (1972), Measuring depression: The depression inventory. In: *Recent Advances in the Psychobiology of the Depressive Illnesses*, eds. T.A. Williams, M.M. Katz & J.A. Shields. Washington, DC: U.S. Government Printing Office, pp. 299-302.

Catell, R.B. (1966), The scree test for the number of factors. *Multivariate Behavioral Research*, 1:140-161.

Centers for Disease Control and Prevention (2003), Cases of HIV infection and AIDS in the United States, 2002. *HIV/AIDS Surveillance Report*, 14:1-40.

Chen, S.Y., Gibson, S., Katz, M.H., Klausner, J.D., Dilley, J.W., Schwarcz, S.K. et al. (2002), Continuing increases in sexual risk behavior and sexually transmitted diseases among men who have sex with men: San Francisco, California, 1999-2001. *American J. Public Health*, 92:1387-1388.

DeVellis, R.F. (1991), *Scale Development: Theory and Applications*. Newbury Park, CA: Sage.

Dilley, J.W., McFarland, W., Woods, W.J., Sabatino, J., Lihatsh, T., Adler, B. et al. (2002), Thoughts associated with unprotected anal intercourse among men at high risk in San Francisco, 1997-1999. *Psychology & Health*, 17:235-246.

Elovich, R. (1995), Harm's way. *The Advocate*, 43:43, May 16.

Gold, R. (1995), Why we need to rethink AIDS education for gay men. *AIDS CARE*, 7(Supplement 1):S11-S19.

Gold, R.S, Skinner, M.J., Grant, P.H. & Plummer, D.C. (1991), Situational factors and thought processes associated with unprotected intercourse in gay men. *J. Acquired Immune Deficiency Syndrome & Human Retrovirology*, 5:259-278.

Halkitis, P.N. (2001), An exploration of perceptions of masculinity in gay men living with HIV. *J. Men's Studies*, 9:413-429.

Halkitis, P.N. & Parsons, J.T. (2003), Intentional unsafe sex (barebacking) among HIV-positive gay men who seek sexual partners on the Internet. *AIDS Care*, 15:367-378.

Halkitis, P.N., Parsons, J.T. & Wilton, L. (2003), Barebacking among gay and bisexual men in New York City: Explanations for the emergence of intentional unsafe behavior. *Archives Sexual Behavior*, 32:351-357.

Halkitis, P.N., Wilton, L., Parsons, J.T. & Hoff, C. (2004), Correlates of sexual risk-taking behavior among HIV seropositive gay men in seroconcordant primary partner relationships. *Psychology, Health, & Medicine*, 9:99-113.

Halkitis, P.N., Wilton, L., Wolitski, R., Parsons, J.T , Hoff, C. & Bimbi, D. (2005), Barebacking identity among HIV-positive gay and bisexual men: Demographic, psychological, and behavior correlates. *AIDS*(Suppl):527-535.

Kalichman, S.C., Kelly, J.A., Morgan, M. & Rompa, D. (1997), Fatalism, current life satisfaction, and risk for HIV infection among gay and bisexual men. *J. Consulting & Clinical Psychology*, 65:542-546.

Kellogg, T, McFarland, W, Perlman, J.L., Weinstock, H., Bock, S., Katz, M.H. et al. (2001), HIV incidence among repeat HIV testers at a county hospital, San Francisco, California, USA. *J. Acquired Immune Deficiency Syndromes*, 28:59-64.

Odets, W. (1995), *In the Shadow of the Epidemic: Being HIV-Negative in the Age of AIDS*. Durham, NC: Duke University Press.

Ostrow, D.G., DiFranceisco, W. & Kalichman, S. (1997), Sexual adventurism, substance use and high risk sexual behavior: A structural modeling analysis of the Chicago MACS/coping and change cohort. *AIDS & Behavior*, 1:191-202.

Shidlo, A. (1994), Internalized homophobia: Conceptual and empirical issues in measurement. In: *Lesbian and Gay Psychology: Theory, Research, and Clinical Applications*, eds. B. Greene & G.M. Herek. Thousand Oaks, CA: Sage, pp. 176-205.

Shidlo, A. (1997), Mental health issues in HIV-negative gay men. In: *HIV Mental Health for the 21st Century*, ed. M. Winiarski. New York: New York University, pp. 173-189.

Shidlo, A. & Dalit, B. (1996), *HIV-Negative Identity in Gay and Bisexual Men: Assessment Issues*. Paper presented at the 18th National Lesbian and Gay Health Conference, Seattle, WA, July 8.

Shidlo, A. & Hollander, G. (1998), *Assessing Internalized Homophobia: New Empirical Findings*. Paper resented at the 106th Annual Convention of the American Psychological Association, San Francisco, CA, August 14.

Suarez, T. & Miller, J. (2001), Negotiating risks in context: A perspective on unprotected anal intercourse and barebacking among men who have sex with men–Where do we go from here? *Archives Sexual Behavior*, 30:287-299.

Tabachnik, B.G. & Fidell, L.S. (1983), *Using Multivariate Statistics*. New York: Harper & Row.

Turner, K.R., McFarland, W., Kellogg, T.A., Wong, E., Page-Shafer, K., Louie, B. et al. (2003), Incidence and prevalence of herpes simplex virus type 2 infection in persons seeking repeat HIV counseling and testing. *Sexual Transmitted Diseases*, 30:331-334.

Victorian AIDS Council (1994), *Relationships: Your Choice*. A publication of the Gay Men's Health Centre, 6 Claremont Street, South Yarra, Victoria 3141, Australia.

Wolitski R.J., Valdiserri, R.O., Denning, P.H. & Levine, W.C. (2001), Are we headed for a resurgence of the HIV epidemic among men who have sex with men? *American J. Public Health*, 91:883-888.

Yalom, I.D. (1995), *Theory and Practice of Group Psychotherapy (4th ed.)*. New York: Basic Books.

Motivating the Unmotivated:
A Treatment Model for Barebackers

Jeffrey T. Parsons, PhD

SUMMARY. Documented increases in sexual risk practices among gay and bisexual men and subsequent increases in HIV infection rates may be attributable, in part, to barebacking. Current HIV prevention efforts fail to meet the needs of diverse gay and bisexual men and do not focus on harm-reduction techniques currently used by such men. Motivational Interviewing (MI), an intervention approach with demonstrated effectiveness across a wide variety of behaviors, may be useful for working with men who bareback. The general principles and strategies of MI are presented with examples of the application of this model to barebacking. *[Article copies available for a fee from The Haworth Document Delivery Service: 1-800-HAWORTH. E-mail address: <docdelivery@ haworthpress.com> Website: <http://www.HaworthPress.com> © 2005 by The Haworth Press, Inc. All rights reserved.]*

Jeffrey T. Parsons is affiliated with the Center for HIV/AIDS Educational Studies and Training (CHEST), the Graduate Center and Hunter College, City University of New York.

Address correspondence to: Jeffrey T. Parsons, PhD, Hunter College, 695 Park Avenue, New York, NY 10021 (E-mail: jeffrey.parsons@hunter.cuny.edu).

The author would like to acknowledge the invaluable assistance of the colleagues that have been instrumental in the development and implementation of Motivational Interviewing interventions targeting gay and bisexual men: Mary Marden Velasquez, Carlo DiClemente, Joseph Carbonari, Jon Morgenstern, Milton Wainberg, Thomas Irwin, Elana Rosof, and Bradley Thomason.

[Haworth co-indexing entry note]: "Motivating the Unmotivated: A Treatment Model for Barebackers." Parsons, Jeffrey T. Co-published simultaneously in *Journal of Gay & Lesbian Psychotherapy* (The Haworth Medical Press, an imprint of The Haworth Press, Inc.) Vol. 9, No. 3/4, 2005, pp. 129-148; and: *Barebacking: Psychosocial and Public Health Approaches* (ed: Perry N. Halkitis, Leo Wilton, and Jack Drescher) The Haworth Medical Press, an imprint of The Haworth Press, Inc., 2005, pp. 129-148. Single or multiple copies of this article are available for a fee from The Haworth Document Delivery Service [1-800-HAWORTH, 9:00 a.m. - 5:00 p.m. (EST). E-mail address: docdelivery@haworthpress.com].

doi:10.1300/J236v09n03_08

KEYWORDS. AIDS, anal sex, barebacking, bisexual men, harm reduction, HIV, homosexuality, intervention, gay men, MSM, motivational interviewing, risk reduction

INTRODUCTION

Gay and bisexual men are reporting more sexual risk behavior than in previous years and there is significant concern that HIV infection rates may once again be on the rise after more than a decade of remaining relatively stable (Catania et al., 2001; Halkitis et al., 2004; Wolitski et al., 2001). Based on the evidence of rising rates of HIV infection among MSM, it is not surprising that recent increases in the rates of sexually transmitted infections (STIs) have been reported in this group of men (Bellis et al., 2002; CDC, 2002; Valdiserri, 2003). See Wolitski in this issue.

These epidemiological findings are consistent with studies documenting an alarming increase in unprotected sexual behaviors among MSM in HIV epicenters with large gay communities (Chen et al., 2002a; Ekstrand et al., 1999; Wolitski et al., 2001). Several factors (i.e., mental health, alcohol/drug use, psychosocial) have been identified as contributing to these increases in both HIV and STIs (Crepaz and Marks, 2002; Wolitski et al., 2001). The recent phenomenon of "barebacking" is one emerging factor that has contributed to increased levels of sexual risk-taking behaviors among MSM (Gauthier and Forsyth, 1999; Goodroad, Kirksey and Butensky, 2000; Halkitis and Parsons, 2003; Halkitis, Parson and Wilton, 2003; Halkitis et al., 2005; Mansergh et al., 2002; Suarez and Miller, 2001).

PROBLEMS WITH EXISTING HIV PREVENTION APPROACHES

Failure to Meet the Needs of Diverse Gay and Bisexual Men

The increases in HIV and STIs among gay and bisexual men point to deficits in current approaches to HIV prevention interventions and counseling programs. Many of the behavioral interventions tested with samples of MSM in the past have been found to be effective (for a review, see Johnson et al., 2002). However, it is often the case that these interventions "preach to the choir." Additional barriers to participation in HIV counseling programs exist. Some HIV preventive interventions fail to address the specific needs of gay and bisexual men, as well as consider carefully the social contexts in which unsafe sexual practices occur. Another relevant factor may involve simple "burnout" from listening to safer sex educational messages and engaging in condom use. It has been suggested that this burnout could lead to a new wave of the HIV epidemic, and it may have already begun (Wolitski et al., 2001).

Other factors may be adversely affecting the effectiveness of existing programs aimed at reducing the spread of HIV among gay and bisexual men. With 20 years of safer sex education, information, and counseling, many of these men have developed complicated risk-management strategies to balance their need for sexual expression with the need for sexual safety. The term "negotiated safety" has been used to describe one of these strategies (Kippax et al., 1993; Van de Ven et al., 2002). Based on the premise of harm reduction, the idea underlying negotiated safety is that two confirmed HIV−men in a committed relationship agree to have unprotected anal sex with each other, but to practice only safer sex outside the relationship. Existing intervention programs may fail to consider these negotiations or fail to carefully explore what sexual activity occurs outside the relationship. It should be noted that these harm-reduction approaches of negotiated safety and strategic sexual positioning are all based on assumptions. In negotiated safety, it is assumed that sex outside the primary relationship involves condom use, as well as the assumption that both members of the couple are in fact HIV−. In strategic sexual positioning, it is assumed that all gay and bisexual men are aware of their HIV status and will position their behavior accordingly. Although negotiated safety and strategic sexual positioning are designed to reduce harm, incorrect assumptions could result in HIV transmission.

Furthermore, the availability, in the past several years, of highly active antiretroviral therapy (HAART) has also been associated with increased sexual risk behaviors, and could be reducing the effectiveness of prevention programs (Dilley, Woods and McFarland, 1997; Kalichman et al., 1998; Kelly et al., 1998; Ostrow et al., 2002; Remien et al., 1998).

Summary

Many current programs and efforts to reduce HIV infection among gay and bisexual may no longer be effective, accounting for some of the recent increases in HIV and STI rates. They may fail to reach the men most at risk, or reach them, but not maintain their involvement. Some men may just be tired of hearing safer sex messages after 20 years. Interventions have not specifically addressed issues such as negotiated safety and strategic sexual positioning, thus ignoring the interpersonal efforts that gay and bisexual men themselves are trying to make in order to stem the epidemic. Nor have prevention programs catering to the gay community explored the impact of new treatments on sexual risk behaviors.

An additional concern is that many existing HIV risk-reduction interventions deemed "effective" through research efforts have *not* been replicated in community-based settings. Many of these programs have been tested in large, well-funded clinical trials, involving many sessions and highly-skilled clinicians. It is questionable whether these interventions can be transferred to and sustained by the gay community. Furthermore, all the existing proven-effective HIV behavioral change programs are aimed at changing behavior in highly motivated individuals who consent to participate. Men who identify themselves as barebackers may be uninterested in such intervention efforts. As such, an intervention approach that could be utilized with gay and bisexual men who bareback, as well as other less motivated persons, is urgently needed as the AIDS epidemic moves into the next phase.

MOTIVATIONAL INTERVIEWING: BACKGROUND

Miller and Rollnick (1991) developed a technique called Motivational Interviewing (MI), which concentrates on the issues of motivation at various points along a continuum of behavior change. The theoretical foundation of MI is grounded in research on the processes of natural recovery and self-change (Sobell and Sobell, 1993). One of the fundamental principles of MI is that individuals naturally have the capacity to find the resources they need to change behavior on their own. MI strategies have been developed that attempt to deal with the resistance, ambivalence, and lack of objective self-assessment that are common, particularly among those in the earlier stages of behavior change (Miller and Rollnick, 1991). These strategies, which include being empathic, "rolling with resistance," emphasizing client choice and responsibility, and avoiding argumentation, have been found to be particularly effective when compared to more confrontational approaches. Clearly, a counselor telling an HIV+ client who barebacks "You just have to start using condoms or you're going to give someone HIV" will have less of a motivating effect than saying "So, you've had difficulty using

condoms in the past, and really like how it feels having sex without them. Let's try to understand what's happening and talk about whether you might want to make some changes in this area." The benefits of using a more supportive, MI approach compared to a directive-confrontational approach has been empirically validated (Miller, Benefield and Tonigan, 1993).

MI methods' impact on motivation of behavior change have been examined in multiple populations, particularly among substance-abusing populations (Bien, Miller and Borough, 1993; Emmons and Rollnick, 2001; Kelly, Halford and Young, 2000; Miller, 1985; Miller and Sovereign, 1989). In Project MATCH, clients who received four MI sessions over a 12-week period attained significant and sustained improvements in drinking outcomes from baseline to one-year post-treatment (Project MATCH Research Group, 1997). Evidence supports the use of MI as a stand-alone treatment for a broad spectrum of drinking problems in both abstinent (Project Match Research Group, 1997) and non-abstinent goal conditions (Miller, 1995). Questions have arisen regarding MI and related treatment methods and whether they demonstrate decreased efficacy over time compared to other treatment methods (Dunn, Deroo and Rivara, 2001). On the other hand, a review by Miller (2000) has shown numerous examples of brief MI sessions that compare favorably with skills training in terms of long-term follow-up. A recent review of MI interventions across a wide spectrum of disorders reached the unexpected conclusion that treatment effects for those in MI conditions did not show significant declines on outcome measures across the length of the follow-up periods (Dunn, Deroo and Rivara, 2001).

One recent study examined the efficacy of MI for marijuana dependence (Stephens, Roffman and Curtin, 2000). It compared two, one-hour sessions of MI as a stand-alone treatment, a 180-hour education intervention, and a waitlist control. Each treatment condition had favorable outcomes compared to the wait-list condition and there were few differences between treatment conditions, in spite of the dramatic difference in client contact. Overall, these findings suggest that MI, delivered as a stand-alone brief intervention, can be effective in treating even those dependent on alcohol or marijuana.

MI has been associated with increased adherence to alcoholism treatment programs (Brown and Miller, 1993) and outpatient substance abuse treatment (Swanson, Pantalon and Cohen, 1999). A recent study integrated MI techniques into a behavioral weight-control program (Smith et al., 1997). Research results showed that, compared to control group participants, participants receiving MI showed significantly greater treatment adherence, including better attendance at group meetings. MI techniques have been found to improve adherence to treatment regimens among diabetics (Trigwell, Grant and House, 1997). In a study of African-American illegal drug users, MI techniques resulted in patients being more involved in the session, more willing to self-disclose, and more likely to seek help for drug-using problems (Longshore, Grills and Annon, 1999). Among opiate abusers, an MI intervention was shown to promote behavior change, increase commitment to change, and reduce likelihood of relapse, compared to an education-only control group (Saunders, Wilkinson and Philips, 1995).

Although MI strategies have been tested less extensively in HIV prevention studies than in substance abuse/dependence treatment studies, there is growing evidence that brief strategies may be just as useful in reducing sexual risk behavior. Carey et al. (1997) developed a brief intervention that incorporated MI strategies and skills training to reduce unprotected sex among low-income urban women. The four-session group intervention significantly reduced unprotected sex in this sample. These results were replicated more recently with similar effect sizes (Carey et al., 2000). A recent study compared a MI and skills intervention with a video-based education control to reduce unsafe sex among heterosexual men (Kalichman, Cherry and Browne, 1999). Both were six hours in length. The results indicated that the MI-skills condition significantly reduced unprotected vaginal intercourse; however, the researchers report that group differences were not significant at six months. MI interventions have also been used as a way of reducing HIV risk behaviors among injection drug users (Baker et al., 1994).

As prevention efforts are shifting back to gay and bisexual men, there has been a recent increase in studies focused on increasing motivation to change sex risk behavior in this population. A recent intervention study found that an MI intervention was effective in reducing HIV risk behaviors among substance abusing MSM (Beadnell et al., 1999) and HIV+ MSM (Fisher and Ryan, 1999). A recent study investigating telephone delivery of MI to reduce HIV risk among MSM suggests that a single session, averaging 90 minutes, reduced unprotected sex among participants compared to participants in a wait-list control condition (Picciano et al., 2001). These results are especially encouraging as they demonstrate that an effective, brief MI intervention, requiring few resources, can be provided to MSM who are not committed to changing sexual risk practices. Harding (2001) combined MI with a cognitive intervention for the purpose of implementing an HIV risk-reduction strategy among

MSM in both commercial venues and environments where public sex occurs. Although outcomes have not yet been tested, these methods allowed for the dissemination of a theoretically based intervention to over 900 men, in settings that have traditionally been very difficult to access by treatment providers.

There are several assumptions inherent in the use of MI. First, motivation is viewed as a state of readiness to change, which may fluctuate from one time or situation to another. The MI approach posits that this state of readiness can be influenced by the counselor. Second, motivation for change does not reside solely within the client. The counselor's style is believed to be a powerful determinant of both client resistance and behavior change. An empathic counseling style is more likely to bring out self-motivational responses and less resistance from the client. Third, people struggling with behavioral problems often have fluctuating and conflicting motivations for change, also known as ambivalence. This ambivalence is a normal part of considering and making change, and is *not* pathological. Finally, the MI approach holds that each client has the potential for change. The task of the counselor is to release that potential and facilitate the natural change process presumed to be inherent in the individual. This is not to imply that MI has empirical support to be 100% successful with all clients; however, the MI approach would resist viewing even the most challenging client as a "hopeless case." MI can best be conceptualized as a style of being with people rather than a set of techniques. There are, however, specific principles and strategies that best fit within the approach.

MOTIVATIONAL INTERVIEWING: GENERAL PRINCIPLES

There are four general guiding principles of MI which are used to engage clients who are ambivalent about making changes to their behavior: (1) expressing empathy, (2) developing discrepancy, (3) rolling with resistance, and (4) supporting self-efficacy (Miller and Rollnick, 1991; 2002).

Expressing Empathy

Regardless of one's own personal feelings about a client's behavior, the counselor should actively listen to the client without communicating any feelings of judgment, criticism, or blame. This will facilitate a better understanding of the client's situations and perspectives. Ideally, em-

pathic communication should be used from the very beginning in interactions with each client. The counselor needs to understand that the
client may not be ready or willing to give up barebacking or change his
sexual practices at the early stages of the process and reluctance to
change should be expected. Thus, the initial focus should be on building
therapeutic rapport and supporting the client instead of directly suggesting change. The key point here is to accept the client where he is at any
given moment. Rather than responding to the barebacking client as if he
were pathological or misbehaving, the counselor should attempt to see
the client's behavior as contextually understandable and comprehensi-
ble. This does not mean that the counselor agrees with or endorses
barebacking behavior. However, by responding to the client's ambivalence about change with comprehension, the client will feel more
comfortable contemplating change in the future.

Developing Discrepancy

One of the goals of MI is to create and amplify discrepancy in the client's mind between their present and past behavior and their future
goals. This can be accomplished through examination of the consequences of continuing a problematic behavior or not adopting a new behavior. Often, a consideration of the *decisional balance* (the pros of
changing and the cons of remaining the same) can facilitate this. Many
men who bareback know the potential risk (both to themselves and to
their sexual partners) that can result from unprotected anal sex. However, they may not have fully considered the costs and benefits of continued barebacking or adopting safer sex practices. The decisional
balance exercise allows for careful consideration of the pros and cons
and also elicits "change talk," which is the client's own expression of
potential change. Here the counselor "directs" the session by selectively
reflecting and summarizing client statements that indicate the client is
moving in the direction of change. The counselor can also use MI skills
to elicit the client's own insight into how his current barebacking behavior is in direct conflict with other important personal goals and values
(i.e., remaining healthy, maintaining positive self-esteem, protecting
others in the gay community). The hope is that the client will eventually
be able to present his own arguments for change. A client who hears
himself arguing for condom use is more likely to change his behavior
than a client who hears his counselor arguing for condom use.

Rolling with Resistance

Typical behavior change approaches can result in the counselor arguing for change and the client arguing against it. This argumentation is not only unproductive, it can actually result in the client becoming more committed to not changing. A client who feels pressured or coerced is likely to express resistance. Sometimes this resistance is expressed through challenging the counselor or denial of a problem. Other times, however, resistance can be expressed as the client giving up. A client who responds to counselor pressure by stating "All right, barebacking is bad and I'll stop" is unlikely to actually accomplish behavior change. MI should not become a contest or a competition between the counselor and the client. Rather than a wrestling match, an MI session has been likened to a dance between the client and counselor (Rollnick, Mason and Butler, 1999). When a counselor is faced with resistance from a client, it becomes important to let the resistance be fully expressed instead of trying to fight against it. The MI approach suggests that a counselor reflect back a client's questions and concerns so that he may further examine the possible alternatives. For example, a counselor could say, "It sounds like you're not sure about changing your barebacking behavior." Thus, the client becomes the source of the possible answers, does not feel defeated in sharing his concerns, and is able to take the risk to express his feelings. Often, resistance is a clear indicator that it is time for the counselor to change strategies.

Supporting Self-Efficacy

Self-efficacy refers to the client's belief in the ability to change his behavior. High self-efficacy is one of the best predictors of behavior change. A counselor can support a client's belief in his ability to change in a variety of ways. One of these is to encourage the client to talk about examples of positive changes that he has made in the past. Another is to emphasize the importance of taking responsibility for one's own behavior. Finally, the client should feel a strong support and a positive rapport with the counselor, which furthers his sense of self-efficacy.

MOTIVATIONAL INTERVIEWING: STRATEGIES

There are five specific strategies which have been found to be useful throughout the MI process in order to address the guiding principles discussed above: (1) asking open-ended questions, (2) affirming, (3) reflective listening, (4) summarizing, and (5) eliciting change talk. It is important to use these strategies starting with the first session, as they are very helpful in assisting clients to explore their ambivalence and clarify their own reasons for behavior change.

Asking Open-Ended Questions

Early in the therapeutic process, it is critical that a trusting and accepting environment be created that allows clients to explore their ambivalence. During the earliest MI sessions, it is more important that the client speak, rather than the counselor. Asking questions that cannot easily be answered with a brief "yes" or "no" or short response will facilitate this. Letting the client do most of the talking helps to establish trust and lets him know the counselor is interested. It also allows the counselor to obtain much information and insight into the client's issues and points to discrepancies between what the client is doing and what he wants to be doing. This is particularly important at the beginning, when the counselor may be unclear as to the client's motivation for change.

A counselor can begin with "What are your thoughts about barebacking?" or "I'd like to understand how you see things going with regard to your sex behaviors. What's brought you here today?" With ambivalent clients, it is important to use open-ended questions to elicit both positive and negative aspects of the problem. For example, it could be useful to first ask a client "Tell me about your barebacking behavior. What are the good things about having sex without condoms?" Then, as a follow-up question, ask about the other side of the issue, "What are your worries about having unprotected sex?" Counselors should be wary, however, of spending too much time on open-ended questions. It has been suggested that in using MI, counselors limit themselves to asking no more than three consecutive questions. The session should not resemble an interrogation, even by keeping the questions open-ended. It is more effective to ask an open-ended question, give the client time to explore their feelings and ambivalence as they respond, and then reflect back what the client has said before moving onto another question.

Affirming

An important strategy in expressing empathy is to affirm and support the client throughout the MI process. This helps to build counselor-client rapport and to reinforce the client's exploration of his own interests in behavior change. Compliments, statements of appreciation and understanding, or just noticing and acknowledging efforts on the part of the client are also effective in enhancing the client's self-efficacy regarding change. Affirming a client for even considering change can be important to affirming maintenance of behavioral change. For example:

> CLIENT: Since I'm not in a relationship, I really want to feel close to the guys I have sex with. I want that feeling of intimacy. And using a condom takes that feeling away.
> COUNSELOR: You really have a lot to offer people, so it's important for you to find ways to express intimacy with others.
> CLIENT: And at the same time, I know if I get an STI, it could make me sick. I've been living with HIV for 15 years now, and I'm still healthy and want to stay that way.
> COUNSELOR: Well, it's clear that you're a very strong person and you're capable of doing whatever it takes to make sure you stay healthy.

Affirming language can be especially important with clients who are less motivated to change. A barebacking client who has few expressed intentions to change still needs to feel affirmed and supported. Otherwise, he may fail to return for additional sessions and the opportunity to explore his ambivalence is lost. Concluding an initial session with, "I really want to thank you for coming in today," "I really enjoyed talking to you and getting to know you better," or "I appreciate how hard it must have been for you to come here today" can be helpful.

Reflective Listening

Reflective listening is sometimes viewed as the most important and difficult strategy in implementing MI. In reflective listening, the counselor guesses at a reasonable meaning behind the client's statement, and articulates this guess in the form of a statement. In using reflective listening, however, what the counselor believes or assumes the client means may not necessarily be what the client actually means. It is also important to reflect the client's words as well as his feelings. Reflections are statements, rather than questions, and as such the inflection in the counselor's voice should go down rather than up. Statements are less likely than questions to trigger resistance because a question usually signals that the counselor is looking for a response on the part of the client.

Reflective statements can be simple, as in repeating the client's exact words. More advanced reflections substitute new words or reflect the counselor's guess as to how the client is feeling. In double sided reflections, conflictual sides of a client's feelngs are reflected, acknowledging that the counselor has heard the client's ambivalence. Reflective listening can also be quite directive as the counselor decides what to emphasize and what to minimize. Further, the counselor can be directive in selecting what specific words and feelings to reflect back to the client. In particular, any statements indicating the client's motivation to change should be reflected back. The following is an example of a client-counselor exchange in which the emphasis is on reflective listening:

CLIENT: You know, I've been barebacking for a long time and nothing bad has happened to me.
COUNSELOR: So, you're not concerned about anything happening to you even though you're barebacking.
CLIENT: Well, I could get infected with HIV, I suppose, but the guys I bareback with are all negative.
COUNSELOR: So you have nothing to worry about.
CLIENT: No, I guess not. Although, it's possible some of the guys I hook up with could be positive.
COUNSELOR: And that worries you.
CLIENT: Well I don't want to get HIV, or syphilis, or anything else for that matter. But, I also don't want to have use condoms every time I want to fuck. The condoms just don't make it feel as good. So, I'm not sure what I want.
COUNSELOR: And you're wondering if maybe you should do something about all this.
CLIENT: I guess so.
COUNSELOR: You're not sure.
CLIENT: I'm not sure what I want to be doing.
COUNSELOR: So, on the one hand, you're concerned about getting infected as a result of barebacking, but on the other hand you want the sex to be as pleasurable as possible, and condoms make sex less enjoyable. So you're not sure yet if you want to make any changes.
CLIENT: Right. It doesn't make a lot of sense does it?
COUNSELOR: I can see how you might feel confused at this point.

Reflective listening is the most critical strategy in expressing empathy and can also be used to affirm the thoughts and feelings of the client.

Reflections can be used effectively to roll with resistance. Sometimes it is useful to amplify reflections by exaggerating what the client has said. This often results in the client backing down from their original thoughts and expressing the other side of their ambivalence.

Summarizing

Summarizing is a form of reflective listening in which the counselor links together and reinforces what has already been discussed. Summarizing should be done periodically throughout a session as a transition to shift the focus. Summary statements are directive, as the counselor chooses which points to summarize. This strategy helps both the counselor and the client stay focused during the session. It also lets a client know he has been heard and helps him elaborate further. Summaries are particularly useful after a client has expressed reasons for changing. For example:

> So, testing positive for gonorrhea last month has really left you feeling conflicted. Although none of the guys you have sex with like using condoms, you're worried about continuing to bareback because next time it could be more than just gonorrhea. You've also mentioned feeling guilty after having bareback sex, and that guilt went up when you realized you could have passed a STI onto some of your sex partners. And, you're concerned about what might happen to your future if you became HIV+ and that continuing to bareback could result in that. What else?

There are three different types of summaries: collecting, linking, and transitional. The example above is a collecting summary of several statements indicating a desire or concern for change expressed by the client. These summaries are typically short and are designed to continue the client's momentum rather than disrupt it. "What else?" or another open-ended question to permit the client to continue should be used to close the collecting summary. Linking summaries are designed to tie together what has been currently discussed with information obtained previously, including information derived in previous MI sessions with the client. These summaries help the client consider the relationship between two or more thoughts. For clients experiencing ambivalence about changing their behavior, a linking summary will help them see both sides simultaneously, as well as showing the client that the counselor sees both sides of the issue. Finally, transitional summaries are used to indicate a shift in focus, again highlighting the directive aspects of MI. At the end of a session, it is useful to offer a major transitional summary that pulls together all that has transpired over the course of the session.

Eliciting Change Talk

The fifth strategy, eliciting change talk, is a major aspect of MI and is designed to help resolve ambivalence. It is where the client tells the counselor the reasons for and advantages of behavior change. However, as MI is a directive style, it is the counselor who makes efforts to elicit change talk from the client. There are four general categories of change talk: (1) recognizing disadvantages of the current situation, (2) recognizing advantages of change, (3) expressing optimism about change, and (4) expressing intention to change. There are several ways in which counselors can elicit change talk from clients. Open-ended evocative questions can be used to explore the client's particular situation. For example:

> What makes you think you need to do something about your barebacking?
> What would be the advantages of using condoms when you have anal sex?
> How confident are you that you can make this change?
> I can see that you're feeling stuck–What's going to have to change?

Another technique commonly used in brief MI interventions (Rollnick, Butler and Stott, 1997; Butler et al., 1999) involves asking the client to rate his motivation to change on a scale of 0 to 10 (0 being low and 10 being high). Then, the counselor can ask the client to explain why they are at that level of motivation and what it would take to get to a higher number. For example:

> COUNSELOR: So, how important would you say it is for you to use condoms every time you have anal sex? On a scale of zero to 10, where zero is not at all important and 10 is extremely important, where would you say you are?
> CLIENT: I really like barebacking and am not sure I want to stop. So, I'd say I'm probably a four.
> COUNSELOR: Why are you at a four and not at a zero?

CLIENT: Well, because sometimes I do get worried that I might infect someone who's negative. Although most guys I bareback with are positive.

COUNSELOR: You would feel guilty if someone else got infected.

CLIENT: Well, yeah. I don't really want to do to someone else what someone did to me.

COUNSELOR: So, you don't want to be responsible for someone else getting HIV infected?

CLIENT: Right.

COUNSELOR: What would it take for you to go from a four to a higher number?

CLIENT: Well, I guess I'd have to find some ways to make sex with a condom more enjoyable.

COUNSELOR: So you don't enjoy having sex when a condom is used.

CLIENT: Well, no. I mean, I enjoy it. It's sex, so on some level you enjoy it. But, it just feels better without a condom.

COUNSELOR: You can enjoy sex if you're using a condom.

CLIENT: Yes, and I know if I put my mind to it, I could bareback less, or make sure I only bareback with other positive guys by disclosing my status. Then, at least, I'd be taking more responsibility. I'm pretty strong-willed when it comes down to something I want.

COUNSELOR: It sounds like you don't want to be responsible for someone else getting HIV and you see yourself as a responsible person. You know that you're capable of having a good time having sex with condoms, and you're very confident that you've got the will power to make this change.

This example shows how change talk can be elicited though the use of the importance question. Specifically, this client expresses disadvantages of the current situation (could infect someone else with HIV and feel guilty), advantages of change (will feel like a responsible person), and optimism about change (he knows he can do it if he puts his mind to it).

Focusing on decisional balance can help to both develop discrepancy and elicit change talk. Having clients describe what they see as the benefits of barebacking, and then subsequently describing the downsides of barebacking can help the client to clarify both aspects of his ambivalence.

It can also be helpful to have the client elaborate on their change talk. When a client presents a reason for change, the counselor should ask for elaboration before moving on. This will both help to generate additional change talk statements and will also serve as a way of affirming and re-inforcing the originally stated motivation for change. Open-ended elaborative questions such as, "In what ways?" or "What else?" may be enough. Counselors can also ask clients to provide specific examples to illustrate their motivational thinking.

Having clients think back to a time before the problem behavior began or having them imagine a time in the future in which they are no longer engaged in the problem behavior can also be useful tools to elicit change talk. In having clients look back, they should be asked to remember the time before they started barebacking (or a time before HIV depending on the client's particular situation) and to compare those times with the current situation. Similarly, having the client to imagine a time in the future when they are not having bareback sex and asking them to describe what they see can be effective. It can also be useful to ask clients to imagine themselves 5 or 10 years in the future if they do not make any changes in their behavior and ask them to describe what might happen.

Throughout the process of eliciting change talk, the client is encouraged to set their own goals with regard to behavior change. As such, it is not necessary for the counselor to impose goals on the client. This permits the client to set realistic and achievable goals without feeling pressured by the counselor. For example, some clients may be ready to set a firm goal such as "I will not bareback anymore." Other clients will set a goal that is more reflective of their current level of motivation to change, such as "I'm going to talk to the partners I have sex with about HIV status before making a decision to bareback." By having the client identify and set their own goals, they take greater ownership over the behavior change process and feel more empowered to take steps to achieve these goals.

CONCLUSIONS

MI has promise as an effective approach to working with gay and bisexual men who engage in barebacking. Following a harm reduction approach, the MI perspective would provide a non-judgmental atmosphere in which clients can explore ambivalence about safer sex practices and HIV/STI infection. By using a directive, client-centered counseling style that enhances motivation for change by helping the client clarify and resolve ambivalence about behavior change, the goal of MI is to create and amplify discrepancy between present behavior and broader goals. It involves listening to, acknowledging, and respecting a broad range of client concerns, beliefs, emotions, and motivations, even when the counselor does not necessarily agree with the client's views.

The client-centered aspect of MI can be used to meet the needs of diverse gay and bisexual men, including those who present with significant motivation to change and those who present with limited motivation. The emphasis on ambivalence can be used to explore how men feel about current harm reduction strategies they are using. And an examination of decisional balance can be utilized to help clients work through lessened concern about contracting and transmitting HIV.

Finally, MI is a way of being with people. We often hear from our clients how much they appreciate coming to see counselors who do not judge them or tell them what to do. When asked what they found helpful about the MI sessions, our clients repeatedly say that they did not feel pressure to change and that the decision to change came from within. For most individuals, this is a new experience.

REFERENCES

Baker, A., Kochan, N., Dixon, J., Heather, N. & Wodak, A. (1994), Controlled evaluation of a brief intervention for HIV prevention among injecting drug users not in treatment. *AIDS Care*, 6:559-570.

Beadnell, B., Rosengren, D., Downey, L., Fisher, D., Best, H., Wickizer, L. & Stielstra, S. (1999), *Motivational Interviewing (MI) to facilitate reduced HIV risk among alcohol using men who have sex with men*. Paper presented at the National HIV Prevention Conference. Atlanta, GA [August 29-September1].

Bellis, M.A., Cook, P., Clark, P., Syed, Q. and Hoskins, A. (2002), Re-emerging syphilis in gay men: A case-control study of behavioural risk factors and HIV status. *J. Epidemiology & Community Health*, 56:235-236.

Bien, T.H., Miller, W.R. & Borough, J.M. (1993), Motivational interviewing with alcohol outpatients. *Behavioral Cognitive Psychotherapy*, 21:347-356.

Brown, J.M. & Miller, W.R. (1993), Motivational interviewing on participation and outcome in residential alcoholism treatment. *Psychology of Addictive Behaviors*, 7:211-218.

Butler, C.C., Rollnick, S., Cohen, D., Russel, I., Bachmann, M. & Stott, N. (1999), Motivational consulting versus brief advice for smokers in general practice: A Randomised trial. *British J. General Practice*, 49:611-616.

Carey, M.P., Maisto, S.A., Kalichman, S.C., Forsyth, A.D., Wright, E.M. & Johnson, B. (1997), Enhancing motivation to reduce the risk of HIV infection for economically disadvantaged urban women. *J. Consulting & Clinical Psychology,* 65: 531-541.

Carey, M.P., Braaten, L.S., Maisto, S.A., Gleason, J.R., Forsyth, A.D., Durant, L.E. & Jaworski, B.C. (2000), Using information, motivational enhancement, and skills training to reduce the risk of HIV infection for low-income urban women: A second randomized clinical trial. *Health Psychology,* 19:3-11.

Catania, J.A., Osmond, D., Stall, R.D., Pollack, L., Paul, J.P., Blower, S. et al. (2001), The Continuing HIV epidemic among men who have sex with men. *American J. Public Health,* 91:907-914.

Centers for Disease Control and Prevention (2002), Unrecognized HIV infection, risk behaviors, and perceptions of risk among young black men who have sex with men–Six U.S. cities, 1994-1998. *Morbidity & Mortality Weekly Report,* 51:733-736.

Chen, S.Y., Gibson, S., Katz, M.H., Klausner, J.D., Dilley, J.W., Schwarcz, S.K. et al. (2002a), Continuing increases in sexual risk behavior and sexually transmitted diseases among men who have sex with men: San Francisco, Calif, 1999-2001. *American J. Public Health,* 92:1387-1388.

Crepaz, N. & Marks, G. (2002), Towards an understanding of sexual risk behavior in people living with HIV: A review of social, psychological, and medical findings. *AIDS,* 16:135-149.

Dilley, J.W., Woods, W. J. & McFarland, W. (1997), Are advances in treatment changing views about high-risk sex? *New England J. Medicine,* 337:501-502.

Dunn, C., DeRoo, L. & Rivara, F.P. (2001), The use of brief interventions adapted from motivational interviewing across behavioral domains. *Addictions,* 96:1774-1775.

Emmons, K. & Rollnick, S. (2001), Motivational interviewing in heath care settings: Opportunities and limitations. *American J. Preventive Medicine,* 20:68-74.

Ekstrand, M.L., Stall, R.D., Paul, J.P., Osmond, D.H. & Coates, T.J. (1999), Gay men report high rates of unprotected anal sex with partners of unknown or discordant HIV status. *AIDS,* 13:1525-1533.

Fisher, D. & Ryan, R. (1999), *The effect of a brief MI-related intervention upon the high-risk sexual practices of HIV+ men.* Paper presented at the National HIV Prevention Conference, Atlanta, GA [August 29-September 1].

Gauthier, D.K. & Forsyth, C.J. (1999), Bareback sex, bug chasers, and the gift of death. *Deviant Behavior,* 20:85-100.

Goodroad, B.K., Kirksey, K.M. & Butensky, E. (2000), Bareback sex and gay men: An HIV prevention failure. *J. Association of Nurses in AIDS Care,* 11:29-36.

Halkitis, P.N., Parsons, J.T. & Wilton, L. (2003), Barebacking among gay and bisexual men in New York City: Explanations for the emergency of intentional unsafe behavior. *Archives Sexual Behavior,* 32:351-357.

Halkitis, P.N. & Parsons, J.T. (2003), Intentional unsafe sex (barebacking) among HIV-positive gay men who seek sexual partners on the Internet. *AIDS Care,* 15:367-378.

Halkitis, P.N., Wilton, L., Parsons, J.T. & Hoff, C. (2004), Correlates of sexual risk-taking behavior among HIV seropositive gay men in seroconcordant primary partner relationships. *Psychology, Health & Medicine,* 9:99-113.

Halkitis, P.N., Wilton, L., Wolitski, R., Parsons, J.T., Hoff, C. & Bimbi, D. (2005), Barebacking identity among HIV-positive gay and bisexual men: Demographic, psychological, and behavior correlates. *AIDS*(Suppl): 527-535.

Johnson, W.D., Hedges, L.V., Ramirez, G., Semaan, S., Norman, L.R., Sogolow, E. et al. (2002), HIV prevention research for men who have sex with men: A Systematic review and meta-analysis. *J. Acquired Immune Deficiency Syndromes*, 30:S118-S129.

Kalichman, S.C., Nachimson, D., Cherry, C. & Williams, E. (1998), AIDS treatment advances and behavioral prevention setbacks: Preliminary assessment of reduced perceived threat of HIV/AIDS. *Health Psychology*, 17:546-550.

Kalichman, S.C., Cherry, C., & Browne, F.C. (1999), Effectiveness of a video-based motivational skills-building HIV risk-reduction intervention for inner-city African American men. *J. Consulting & Clinical Psychology*, 67:959-966.

Kelly, A.B., Halford, W.K. & Young, R. (2000), Martially distressed women with alcohol problems: The impact of a short-term alcohol-focused intervention on drinking behaviour and marital satisfaction. *Addiction*, 95:1537-1549.

Kelly, J.A., Hoffman, R.G., Rompa, D. & Gray, M. (1998), Protease inhibitor combination therapies and perceptions of gay men regarding AIDS severity and the need to maintain safer sex. *AIDS*, 12:91-95.

Kippax, S., Crawford, J., Davis, M., Roddin, P. & Dowsett, G. (1993), Sustaining safer sex: A longitudinal study of a sample of homosexual men. *AIDS*, 7:257-263.

Longshore, D., Grills, C. & Annon, K. (1999), Effects of a culturally congruent intervention on cognitive factors related to drug-use recovery. *Substance Use & Misuse*, 34:1223-1241.

Mansergh, G., Marks, G., Colfax, G., Guzman, R., Rader, M. & Buchbinder, S. (2002), Barebacking in a diverse sample of men who have sex with men. *AIDS*, 16:653-659.

Miller, W.R. (1985), Motivation for treatment: A review with special emphasis on alcoholism. *Psychological Bulletin*, 98:84-107.

Miller, W.R. (1995). Increasing motivation for change. In: *Handbook of Alcoholism Treatment Approaches: Effective Alternatives*, eds. R.K. Hester & W.R. Miller. Boston: Allyn and Bacon, pp. 89-104.

Miller, W.R. (2000), Rediscovering fire: Small interventions, large effects. *Psychology of Addictive Behaviors*, 14:6-18.

Miller, W.R. & Sovereign, R. (1989), The check up: A model for early intervention in addictive behaviors. In: *Addictive Behaviors: Prevention and Early Intervention*, eds. P. Nathan & G. Marlatt. Amsterdam: Smets and Zeitlinger.

Miller, W.R. & Rollnick, S. (1991), *Motivational Interviewing: Preparing People to Change Addictive Behavior*. New York: Guilford Press.

Miller, W.R. & Rollnick, S. (2002), *Motivational Interviewing: Preparing People for Change. 2nd Edition*. New York: Guilford Press.

Miller, W.R., Benefield, R.G. & Tonigan, J.S. (1993), Enhancing motivation for change in problem drinking: A Controlled comparison of therapist styles. *J. Consulting & Clinical Psychology*, 61:455-461.

Ostrow, D.E., Fox, K.J., Chimel, J.S., Silvestre, A., Visscher, B.R., Vanable, P.A. et al. (2002), Attitudes towards highly active antiretroviral therapy are associated with sexual risk taking among HIV-infected and uninfected homosexual men. *AIDS*, 16:775-780.

Picciano, J.F., Roffman, R.A., Kalichman, S.C., Rutledge, S.E. & Berghuis, J.P. (2001), A telephone based brief intervention using motivational enhancement to facilitate HIV risk reduction among MSM: A pilot study. *AIDS & Behavior*, 5:251-262.

Project Match Research Group, (1997), Matching alcoholism treatments to client heterogeneity: Project MATCH posttreatment drinking outcomes. *J. Studies on Alcohol*, 58:7-29.

Remien, R.H., Wagner, G., Carballo-Dieguez, A. & Dolezal, C. (1998), Who may be engaging in high-risk sex due to medical treatment advances? *AIDS*, 12:1560-1561.

Rollnick, S., Mason, P. & Butler, C. (1999), *Health Behavior Change: A Guide for Practitioners*. London: Churchill Livingstone.

Rollnick, S., Butler, C.C. & Stott, N. (1997), Helping smokers make decisions: The enhancement of brief intervention for general medical practice. *Patient Education & Counseling*, 31:191-203.

Saunders, B., Wilkinson, C. & Phillips, M. (1995), The impact of a brief motivational intervention with opiate users attending a methadone programme. *Addiction*, 90: 415-424.

Smith, D.E., Heckmeyer, C.M., Kratt, P.P. & Mason, D.A. (1997), Motivational interviewing to improve adherence to a behavioral weight-control program for older obese women with NIDDM. *Diabetes Care*, 20:52-54.

Sobell, M.B. & Sobell, L.C. (1993), *Problem Drinkers: Guided Self-Change Treatment*. New York: Guilford Press.

Stephens, R.S., Roffman, R.A. & Curtin, L. (2000), Comparison of extended versus brief treatments for marijuana use. *J. Consulting & Clinical Psychology*, 68: 898-908.

Suarez, T. and Miller, J. (2001), Negotiating risks in context: A perspective on unprotected anal intercourse and barebacking among men who have sex with men–Where do we go from here? *Archives Sexual Behavior*, 30:287-300.

Swanson, A.J., Pantalon, M.V. & Cohen, K.R. (1999), Motivational interviewing and treatment adherence among psychiatric and dually diagnosed patients. *J. Nervous & Mental Disorders*, 187(10):630-635.

Trigwell, P., Grant, P.J. & House, A. (1997), Motivation and glycemic control in diabetes mellitus. *J. Psychosomatic Research*, 43:307-315.

Valdisseri, R. (2003), *Preventing New HIV Infections in the U.S.: What Can We Hope to Achieve?* Paper presented at the 10th Conference on Retroviruses and Opportunistic Infections: Boston, MA, February.

Van de Ven, P., Kippax, S., Crawford, J., Rawstorne, P., Prestage, G., Grulich, A. et al. (2002), In a minority of gay men, sexual risk practice indicates strategic positioning for perceived risk reduction rather than unbridled sex. *AIDS Care*, 14:471-480.

Woltiski, R.J., Valdiserri, R.O., Denning, P.H. & Levine, W.C. (2001), Are we headed for a resurgence in the HIV epidemic among men who have sex with men? *American J. Public Health*, 91:883-888.

Condomless Sex:
Considerations for Psychotherapy
with Individual Gay Men and Male
Couples Having Unsafe Sex

Michael Shernoff, MSW

SUMMARY. This article explores a variety of interpersonal, intra-psychic, and communal dynamics that have an impact on gay men's safer sex practices. Therapists working with gay men who have condomless sex can have a greater influence in helping them to facilitate change and to understand the meaning of their behavior. This can be done through a non-judgmental and harm reduction approach which eschews holding preconceived ideas about how gay men should conduct their sexual lives. Depression, loneliness, intimacy, HIV status, substance abuse, and love may influence gay men's choices about sex. Using clini-

Michael Shernoff is in Private Practice in Manhattan and Adjunct Faculty, Columbia University School of Social Work. Author and editor of numerous books and articles, he can be reached via his web site www.gaypsychotherapy.com.

The author would like to thank the following individuals for their generosity in reading and providing insights, suggestions, and valuable feedback on early drafts of this article: Michael Bettinger, PhD; John Goodman; Laura Morrision; Robert Remien, PhD and Gil Tunnell, PhD. Additionally, Tim Horn was invaluable in helping locate pertinent references.

[Haworth co-indexing entry note]: "Condomless Sex: Considerations for Psychotherapy with Individual Gay Men and Male Couples Having Unsafe Sex." Shernoff, Michael. Co-published simultaneously in *Journal of Gay & Lesbian Psychotherapy* (The Haworth Medical Press, an imprint of The Haworth Press, Inc.) Vol. 9, No. 3/4, 2005, pp. 149-169; and: *Barebacking: Psychosocial and Public Health Approaches* (ed: Perry N. Halkitis, Leo Wilton, and Jack Drescher) The Haworth Medical Press, an imprint of The Haworth Press, Inc., 2005, pp. 149-169. Single or multiple copies of this article are available for a fee from The Haworth Document Delivery Service [1-800-HAWORTH, 9:00 a.m. - 5:00 p.m. (EST). E-mail address: docdelivery@haworthpress.com].

149

cal case examples, therapeutic strategies for working with individual gay men and couples are discussed. *[Article copies available for a fee from The Haworth Document Delivery Service: 1-800-HAWORTH. E-mail address: <docdelivery@haworthpress.com> Website: <http://www.HaworthPress. com> © 2005 by The Haworth Press, Inc. All rights reserved.]*

KEYWORDS. AIDS, barebacking, condomless sex, gay men, harm reduction, high risk sex, HIV, homosexuality, male couples, MSM, unprotected anal intercourse, unsafe sex

INTRODUCTION

Although none of my gay male psychotherapy patients who have unsafe sex have ever referred to themselves as "bug chasers" (HIV-negative gay men who actively try to get infected), or "gift givers" (HIV-positive gay men who are willing to knowingly infect others), a tour of chat rooms where gay men cruise for sex reveals that these terms are currently used with alarming regularity. Several of my psychotherapy patients who engage in sex that can transmit HIV seek out partners on the Internet. In chat rooms, countless men advertise a desire to "bareback," which refers to having anal sex without a condom. According to Remien and Stirratt (2002), "The most important characteristics of 'barebacking' are the intentionality of condomless sex–as opposed to unprotected sex resulting from poor planning, 'relapse' into risk after consistent condom use, accidents, etc." (p. 2).

An article from a national gay and lesbian newsmagazine referred to Internet chat rooms as "the new gay bars" (Fries, 1998). Several studies conducted both in the United States and Europe have shown that people who use the Internet to meet sexual partners have increased levels of high risk behaviors (Elford, Bolding and Sherr, 2001; Halkitis and Parsons, 2003; Halkitis, Parsons and Wilton, 2003a; McFarlane, Bull and Fietmeijer, 2000; Kim, Kent and McFarland, 2001). Many of the factors that contribute to "cyber cruising" (using the Internet to find sexual partners) foster high-risk sex. For example, psychosocial factors such as depression, antigay violence, childhood sexual abuse, and substance abuse have been shown to have an impact on gay men's sexual risk-taking behaviors (Osborne, 2002). Loneliness, HIV status, unmet intimacy needs, feeling alienated from the gay community, and love are other factors that need to be considered.

Significant numbers of gay men have online profiles stating they are "chem friendly" or want to "party," indicating a desire to have sex while using methamphetamine (i.e., speed, crystal meth, crystal or Tina), GHB, "ecstasy" or other "party drugs." Research demonstrates that high risk behaviors that spread HIV and other STIs occur more frequently among individuals who have poor impulse control, particularly if their sexual activity takes place under the influence of alcohol or drugs (Chesney, Barrett and Stall, 1998; Halkitis and Parsons, 2002; Halkitis, Parsons and Wilton, 2003b; Leigh, 1990; Royce et al., 1997; Stall and Leigh, 1994; Stall et al., 1986; Stall et al., 1991). Regardless of HIV status, many men in my practice who use the Internet to find sexual partners report that they use these terms to locate organized sex parties and/or individuals for a sexual liaison.

It would be simplistic to adduce a single issue or dynamic as the "reason" for an individual's engagement in unsafe sex. Usually a complex combination of factors underlies such behavior, some of which might be otherwise understandable and adaptive for that particular individual. Theories abound as to the resurgence of unsafe sex among gay men: "When we discuss the issue of sexual risk-taking behaviors–particularly in a marginalized, outlawed group, such as gay men–it is imperative to see the historical and cultural forces at work in shaping dynamic understanding of such behavior. No gay man grows up immune to the insidious and overt messages that his sexual desire is in itself fundamentally wrong and unacceptable" (Forstein, 2002, p. 39). Further, Cheuvront (2002) wisely cautions: "In marginalizing the risk-taker as a damaged other, anxieties and fears about risk of infection are quelled for patients and clinicians alike. However, when risk-taking behavior is seen as situational, treatment provides a context for inquiry, articulation and understanding of the patient's unique experiences, feelings and circumstances" (p. 12).

When gay men opt to have high-risk sex, the onset of combination HIV antiretroviral therapy is sometimes a contributing factor (Kelly, Hoffman and Rompa, 1998; Remien and Smith, 2000). Remien and Stirratt (2002) report that complacency about HIV and AIDS, as connected to the development of combination antiretroviral therapy, has resulted in some gay men taking greater risks due to "safer sex burnout." In the early days of the AIDS epidemic, fear propelled men to change how they had sex, since whenever one ventured into a gay neighborhood, critically ill people with AIDS were ubiquitous. Today, highly active antiretroviral therapy (HAART), improved prophylaxis, and weight training (in combination with testosterone, human growth hormone, and steroids) have had a major impact on the physicality of people living HIV and AIDS (Halkitis, 2000; Shernoff, 2002). Without visual reminders, even gay men who are well informed about the transmission of HIV and how it is transmitted are more likely to take sexual risks. As Roberto,[1] a 29 year-old attorney explained:

> I know intellectually this is wrong, but today AIDS just does not seem to be a big deal. I hear from my gay uncle who is in his 50s that in the early days of the epidemic it was pretty common to see prematurely aged gay men in wheel chairs, or covered with lesions, or who looked like they had just come out of Dachau. I have never knowingly seen anyone who was seriously ill with AIDS. I guess this contributes to why I am not as afraid of getting HIV as I should be and why I am not always careful sexually.

One rationalization for engaging in unsafe sex is the belief that having an HIV infection might lessen worry about becoming infected. Such was the case for Mathew, a 36-year-old Wall Street professional whose anxiety was interfering with his very demanding job. He was conservative about sexual risk-taking to the point that his unwillingness to tongue-kiss brought several promising relationships to an end. In his first therapy session, Matthew said he had sought therapy because he felt that, as a sexually active gay man, it was inevitable that he would become infected with HIV and often took sexual risks. "That way, once it happens, I will no longer obsess about whether or not I am infected." Feeling there were better ways for him to learn to control his anxiety, concurrent with his therapy, I referred him to a psycho-pharmacologist.

POWER AND VULNERABILITY

Recent research has demonstrated that some men in known serodiscordant (one HIV+ and one HIV− partner) relationships have high risk sex (Remien et al., 1995; Remien et al., 2001). For example, Remien and his colleagues report that men in serodiscordant couples perceive the risk to be an expression of intimacy, closeness, love and commitment, and that often it is the uninfected partner who pushes for increased levels of sexual risk-taking. The following case illustrates how unsafe sex was used by a younger man in an effort to address his own sense of powerlessness and vulnerability within a relationship with an older, more affluent man who was not as invested in the relationship. The dynamic of using sex as a commodity for barter within a relationship–whether consciously or unconsciously–is obviously not limited to same sex relationships. But, when the aspect of sex that is offered as barter is unprotected anal intercourse by an HIV-negative man in a serodiscordant relationship, the emotional and physical implications become increasingly complex.

Joe, a 30-year-old white HIV-negative gay man originally entered therapy to deal with having an alcoholic and violent father. He has a history of depression largely controlled by antidepressants. During the third year of therapy, Joe courted and began a relationship with Adolph, a prominent health care professional within the gay community who was a decade older. On their first date, Adolph shared that he was an HIV-positive, long-term non-progressor. Joe was not concerned since they agreed about what precautions they would take sexually.

The relationship was problematic from the beginning, as Joe felt he was much more in love with Adolph than Adolph ever was with him. This made Joe feel insecure and sad, especially since he considered Adolph to be a "catch," even though Adolph was still mourning the death of a lover who had died several years earlier. About six months into the relationship, Joe reported that while he was the inserter during anal intercourse, he pulled out, took the condom off, and continued until both partners had each reached orgasm. In discussing what had just occurred, both partners felt excited and concerned. Neither of the men considered the "top" position in unprotected anal intercourse with an HIV-positive man to be completely free of risk, even if the receptive partner's viral loads were below the level of detectability.

In his therapy, Joe said that in addition to the improved sensation condomless sex provided, it also made him feel more spontaneous. Urged to delve deeper into what motivated this behavior, he described having researched available medical literature. Despite having found a few medical journal articles that reported the presence of HIV in the semen of positive men with undetectable levels in their blood, he felt this was low-risk to him. Since he had been thinking about this enough to do the research, what had prevented him from discussing the matter in therapy? He described feeling ashamed and embarrassed about wanting to have unprotected sex, and fearful of what my reaction would be. I said it seemed as if he might be projecting his own ambivalence about having unsafe sex onto me. Joe concurred with this observation and communicated that he had not actually planned on when he would stop using a condom. Since he and Adolph had not discussed it in advance, it was an impulsive behavior and something he needed to continue to explore.

Joe entered one session visibly uncomfortable. When asked why, he responded: "Over the weekend, while Adolph had been fucking me, I thought if he took off the condom, it would feel better, and I would feel closer to him. So I told him to take it off. Adolph complied, continued, but then withdrew before orgasm." Afterwards they both shared how hot this had been but how nervous it made them. Using Joe's stated hope that having anal intercourse without a condom would help him feel closer to Adolph as a starting point, I began to talk about what had occurred. Joe communicated that he did not feel as close to Adolph as he wanted. As Joe began to cry, he reported feeling desperate about wanting to make the relationship work. Their relationship remained rocky, and they even broke up once during an earlier weekend trip. Despite having not used condoms, Joe sensed a reluctance on Adolph's part to allow their relationship to grow. Adolph appeared to have no interest in having Joe move into his large apartment, despite their spending almost every night there together for over eighteen months.

As tensions with Adolph escalated, Joe became depressed. They continued to have unprotected anal sex with Adolph withdrawing prior to orgasm. After a follow-up HIV test confirmed that Joe remained uninfected, he called for an emergency session. Instead of feeling relieved, Joe reported feeling despondent and even more desperate. He said that no matter what he did to try and please Adolph, he always wound up feeling the way he did as a child when his father was drinking and completely unavailable to him. He recognized that part of his attraction to Adolph had been his fantasy of having this older, attractive man take care of him and love him in a way that he had never experienced from his father. He realized now that this would never happen. When asked what he thought the solution was, without skipping a beat, he said: "I need to get out of this before I do something even crazier than I have been doing." He proceeded to talk about his feelings regarding having unsafe sex more deeply than he had ever before. Every time he and Adolph had unprotected sex, he felt badly about himself and worse about the relationship. He was angry that Adolph had gone along with his suggestions of not using condoms. By the following session, Joe had ended their relationship. Although feeling sad, Adolph was not greatly distressed, and he did not try to convince Joe to reconsider. This confirmed Joe's confidence in his decision. Within a week of the break-up, Joe's depression began to lessen.

In the sessions that followed, Joe reported that what he felt Adolph most valued in him was his youth and sexual energy. He had hoped that by not using condoms–and by offering Adolph something unique and special within the sexual realm of their relationship–that Adolph's feelings for him would grow. Joe described that historically, he felt most strong, powerful and in control only during sexual encounters where his partner expressed a strong intensity of desire for him, and often doubted that he had anything else to offer a potential partner. This was as true during recreational sexual encounters as when he was seriously dating someone. As he began to recognize that Adolph was not deeply interested in him beyond their sexual connection, he felt that engaging in unsafe sex was the only option open to him to get Adolph to see how special he was. When unprotected anal intercourse failed to deepen their relationship, Joe was devastated, and found himself sinking into depression. He was confronted with his own longings to be seen as something more than a "hot, young sexual commodity," both by himself and by the men with whom he partnered. The end of the relationship with Adolph was an opportunity to begin to explore this issue in depth.

Joe's case illustrates how high-risk sex can be a means of attempting to ameliorate feelings of powerlessness and helplessness and may appear to the sexual risk taker to be an adaptive option. Clearly, Joe's family history and depression contributed to his decision to place himself in a potentially risky situation, as so much of his sense of self-worth was bound up in confusing feeling sexually desirable with being loved and valued for he was as a whole person.

DEPRESSION AND LONELINESS

For many lonely and isolated gay men, whether depressed or not, protected and or unprotected sex is often an attempt to numb feelings of sadness, boredom, depression, loneliness, and isolation. While symptoms of depression can include low energy or fatigue that can translate into a loss of sex drive, some depressed people become hyperactive sexually (American Psychiatric Association, 2002) and sometimes engage in behaviors that can spread HIV. While these dynamics and characterizations are not true for all sexual risk-takers, for some it is an accurate representation. Other depressed individuals have reported that, as gay men, it was a virtual certainty that they would eventually become HIV infected, and said this was why they never bothered to take sexual precautions. As the following case illustrates, when individuals use "recreational" drugs as a means of self-medication for their depression and anxieties, the likelihood of their taking precautions to prevent HIV transmission is greatly decreased.

Robert is an attractive, 47-year-old African-American HIV-positive gay man who sought therapy to address his crystal methamphetamine use. He grew up in a middle-class, Catholic family in the Midwest. His great passion as a child was figure skating, and he became a regional champion while in high school. Robert knew that he was gay from a young age, and at 15 he discovered a park near his home where he would meet men for sex. These sexual experiences coincided with his beginning to use marijuana and hallucinogenic drugs. He was an above average student who always felt alone and different from other children, even his siblings. "Those moments when men were paying attention to me, either cruising me or while we were having sex, were the only times I ever felt any sort of connection to anyone outside of my family, as fleeting as that connection was."

After college, Robert moved to Manhattan to begin a successful career. He became active in New York's gay party scene, "My entire social life revolved around the five D's: Drugs, Disco, Dick, Dishing, and Dining, in that order." Robert has always wanted but never had a serious boyfriend and described symptoms of a life-long depression. He was amenable to a psychiatric consultation, which resulted in him beginning an antidepressant medication. It was suggested to Robert that if he wanted to reduce or stop drug use, he would have to find people with whom to socialize who did not use drugs. Since his social life entirely revolved around people who used drugs, when Robert did not go out on weekends, he became socially isolated and very lonely. He was adamant in his refusal to attend twelve-step meetings, but he did join a group for newly sober men run by the substance use program in a gay community center.

Although extremely attractive and gregarious in professional venues, Robert felt shy, insecure, and unattractive in gay social situations: "Abstractly, chatting with other men on the Internet seemed like such a safe and innocuous way to pass the time. That is until it immediately became clear that everyone was cruising for sex. So, instead of meeting someone at a club when we were both already high and then going home to do more drugs and carry on, I found myself spending entire weekends doing crystal and having sex. My profile clearly stated that I was HIV-positive, but that never seemed to matter to any of the guys I played with once we got high. Sure, I felt badly about not using condoms. But, I figured that since they knew that I was Poz, they must also be since never once did any of them raise the issue of playing safely. Had anyone mentioned condoms, I certainly would have used them."

Early in treatment, Robert was unable to stay drug free for more than a few weeks. He cited boredom and loneliness as his reasons for calling friends to get high and go dancing or for going online. Both activities ended in unsafe sex. In exploring options for alternative ways to spend time that would be sober and interesting, Robert came up with the idea of training to compete in the Gay Games as a figure skater. So it would not be an isolating activity, he found a partner with whom to train and compete in the ice-dancing category. His commitment to train early in the morning and on weekends helped him stay drug free for longer periods of time. Robert realized that it was impossible for him to be on the ice and safely lift a partner if he was crashing off crystal.

In addition, as Robert said he lacked spirituality in his life, I suggested he attend mass at a local Catholic parish that welcomed gay and lesbian people. This made him feel socially insecure about not knowing how to "homosocialize." I encouraged him to stay after mass for the coffee hour and we role-played how to initiate conversations with people that were not sexual come-ons. This was a slow process that eventually led to his being asked to go out for brunch with other gay men after Mass.

As Robert's life became more balanced, he spent less time on the Internet. He loved to dance and party and did not want to stop completely. Since his goal was to limit the amount of drugs he used, I adopted a "harm reduction" approach with him (Springer, 1991). Robert loved attending circuit parties–multi-day dance parties attended by thousands of gay men–where there is a high level of drug use and sexual activity and a high risk for transmitting HIV (Colfax et al., 2001; Mattison et al., 2001). He had not attended any of these events during the first year of therapy and planned to attend an upcoming gay Disney event in Florida. Robert discussed using drugs but limiting this to small quantities of methamphetamine and ecstasy; he also planned to bring condoms and have only safer sex.

Upon returning home, Robert was pleased he had stuck to his plan, having used methamphetamine only one night. He met someone with whom he partied throughout the weekend. Robert had told this man he was HIV-positive before they left the dance floor, and they used condoms for anal sex. In contrast with his previous drug and sex binges, Robert was not depressed and physically wrung-out for five days afterwards. He and the man he met made plans to get together in New York a few weeks later. They spoke on the phone and via e-mail daily since each returned home. Robert felt excited about learning to date for the first time in his life, even if it was long distance. He relished the conversations and e-mails during which he and his new friend got to know one another in a non-sexual yet romantic way. During the visit by Robert's friend to New York, they did a small amount of drugs and did not have high-risk sex. That visit was the last time Robert and this sexual partner got together. Although Robert was sad and disappointed, he did not use chat rooms for about four months; when he utilized the chat rooms, it was for a sexual liaison part of which was in connection with the use of a small amount of drugs and condoms for anal sex.

When home alone with unstructured time, Robert did not feel desperate. He attributed this to his antidepressant medication. He no longer felt that he was a loser who would never make friends nor have a boyfriend. This change had come about primarily through his affiliation with the church and with his skating partner who was including him in social activities. Guss (2000) suggests that when doing therapy with gay men who abuse Crystal, it is wise to counsel them that sex will never be as intense as it was while they were using drugs. Having employed this strategy with Robert, he said that my making him aware that sober sex would never compare to sex while high had been crucial in establishing my credibility in his eyes, "You did not bullshit me about how sober sex could ever be like what sex on crystal was."

Early in our work, Robert had been nervous that I might try to pressure him to abstain from drugs completely. He knew he was unwilling or unable to do this. Had I pushed for abstinence, Robert would not have remained in therapy for very long. Instead, we discussed his plans to attend three or four circuit parties a year, and to continue limiting his use of drugs to small quantities. He has stuck with this regime for over a year. When Robert used drugs, the use of smaller quantities helped him not to get caught up in the heat of a sexual moment and cease to care about having protected sex. After two years, Robert terminated therapy with the feeling that he had developed a few friendships. However, more importantly, he was learning how to make more friends and date. His drug use was not out of control and he always had safer sex.

The work with Robert is an important reminder that therapy begins by joining with an individual at his starting point and exploring both his desire as well as his capacities for change. Robert's problem at work as a result of his drug use brought him into treatment but was not identified by him as a "problem" for many months. It became clear to Robert that my therapeutic goals did not include trying to convince him to stop using drugs, online sexual hookups, or unprotected anal intercourse–unless he felt ready to so. Only when I had earned enough trust could I gently push him to examine how he felt about each of these activities, as well as what each of them meant to him. Furthermore, the use of antidepressants in ameliorating many of his depressive symptoms provided him with the psychic resilience necessary to tolerate the discomfort that accompanied exploring each of these issues.

COUPLES AND UNSAFE SEX

Male couples living in the age of AIDS need to balance different desires, sexual tastes, and levels of comfort regarding what risk taking, if any, is acceptable. How these issues are raised, discussed, and negotiated are indications of the emotional climate created in the couple's daily interactions and shared emotional life. Research confirms that both HIV-concordant and HIV-discordant male couples are having unprotected sex (Halkitis et al., 2004; Hoff et al., 1997). Men in HIV-concordant relationships reported significantly higher rates of unprotected anal intercourse than discordant couples (Hoff et al., 1997). Remien (1997) discusses the relationship between communication and risk behaviors in serodiscordant couples and the need for therapeutic interventions for couples around these issues Therapists working with male couples must inquire about whether the couple is having safer sex. Inquiring how the men arrived at their decision and how each feels about the level of sexual safety they practice will illuminate dynamics of their communication styles and issues related to power, control, and emotional safety.

Michael and Burt are two HIV-negative gay men in their mid-thirties, who had been a couple for three years and had recently bought an apartment together. They sought couples therapy to discuss the possibility of stopping the use of condoms since they had been monogamous for the past two years. Each had retested negative for HIV in the past two weeks. Michael explained that he began pressuring Burt to agree explicitly to be sexually exclusive after they had been dating for six months. This coincided with first telling each other that they loved one another. Hearing this, Burt explained, "While I knew I had fallen in love with Michael and wanted to spend my life with him, when he first raised the monogamy issue it just felt wrong. It was too soon. Even though I was not having sex with other men, I did not want to make a promise that I did not feel ready to keep. It felt like too much pressure. I wasn't ready to trust him that much at that time. Now it is different."

Michael stated that one of the primary reasons he wanted a monogamous relationship with another HIV-negative man was so that they could forget about safer sex. Neither had ever had anal sex without a condom, nor experienced anyone ejaculating in their mouths, both of which excited them. Each felt that being in a sexually exclusive relationship with a man he loved provided the perfect opportunity to expand his sexual boundaries. "Having that latex barrier between us seems like such a metaphor for our love and relationship not being able to grow any stronger or closer," Burt said.

Each of them were asked if he was willing to trust the other, since there were potential high risks for HIV. The couple provided almost identical responses. They had purchased their apartment and merged their finances, which involved an extremely high level of trust in one another and in the relationship. They also had a realistic understanding of the potential limits of monogamy. The couple was confident that if either partner did have sex outside the relationship, then it would be a serious issue but would not necessarily bring the partnership to an end. Did their definition of monogamy involve having sex together with another person or with other people? At this point, both partners became noticeably uncomfortable. Asked about this, in an uncharacteristically timid manner, Michael responded: "Are we monogamous if we occasionally have played together with another guy?" I asked if they had already done that and both nodded. I responded, "The rules and definitions of your sexual relationship are up to you to decide. But, this raises an important issue about safer sex that we need to talk about."

I explained the concept of "negotiated safety" (Kippax et al., 1993; Prestage et al., 1994) as an agreement between two gay men in a relationship to have a process of getting ready to stop using condoms when they have anal sex. The basis of this agreement is an explicit understanding that both know each other's HIV status and are both uninfected. If they decided to incorporate a "negotiated safety" protocol into their relationship, then they would not just be agreeing to have anal sex with each other without condoms; in addition, the couple would be agreeing to make a serious effort to make anal sex without condoms as safe as possible for both of them. I stressed that such an understanding would be based upon their knowing each other well enough to deal with difficult situations together. For example, if one of them should have unprotected sex outside the relationship, then it would only work if they had complete trust in one another. Previously during anal sex, it was the condom that had provided protection from HIV, and that if they agreed not to use condoms, only their agreement would be protecting them. In other words, the agreement would have to be strong. Four additional sessions were spent talking through all of their feelings about this, and they ultimately decided to forego using condoms. At a follow-up session, eighteen months later, they reported having completely unprotected sex with each other, as well as occasional "play sessions" with other men, which were very safe. They had retested HIV-negative and were thrilled with the arrangement: "It's great that we have all these special sexual treats that we only indulge in with each other. Yet, we also enjoy a bit of safer sexual variety," Michael explained.

Jake and Mark are two healthy HIV-positive gay men in their 50s. Each of the men had lost a previous lover to AIDS. Neither partner had a detectable level of HIV. The couple had been together for two years when they came in for a consultation, prior to moving in together. They had concerns about how this change would impact them individually and as a couple. It was clear that they loved each other deeply and had a rich, interesting, and sensual partnership, which was sexually exclusive.

The couple wanted to explore relaxing their stringency about safer sex. "I really want to drink him," Mark said. "Since we are each undetectable, there is no way we can test to see if we have the same strain of the virus. I love him more than I have ever loved any of my previous partners. Being able to drink his semen is a form of spiritual communion for me. It would make me feel even closer to him than I already do." Jake: "I am not comfortable with the even low level of possibility that I might be giving this man who I adore something that could negatively have an impact on his health, even though he is willing to accept that risk." Mark shared that he also wanted not to use condoms for anal sex. When Mark was questioned about changing their sexual status quo, he said that if Jake wanted to use a condom for anal sex, despite preferring how anal sex felt without one, he could live with that. Mark explained that they were both middle-aged men who were already HIV-infected and had lived more than a decade longer than either had expected. He did not see what difference it would make in the long run to his health, even if Jake gave him a different strain of the virus. As they struggled with trying to decide whether to have unsafe sex, they were also considering whether to open up their sexual relationship for an occasional *menage-a-trois*. Both partners felt strongly that prior to risking a "three way," they would disclose their HIV statuses to any potential sexual partners and would not have no anal sex without a condom.

Mark did not appear either depressed, impulsive, or self-destructive. He understood that there was some possibility of becoming reinfected with another strain of HIV. He was conversant with the medical literature currently debating the entire issue of HIV reinfection, which in the current medical terminology is labeled HIV superinfection.[2] Jake was sufficiently emotionally autonomous that it seemed unlikely he would feel obliged to engage in behavior with which he was uncomfortable. Drugs were not a big part of their lives, although on occasion, they smoked marijuana or had a drink.

Eventually recognizing how much it meant to Mark to receive his semen, Jack decided he would try to become more comfortable with this situation. He feared he might lose his erection if he did not pull out prior to ejaculating, and for a short time after not using condoms, he indeed occasionally did. This was not a major concern for either of them, and it very quickly ceased to occur. Before stopping therapy, they began to ejaculate in each other's mouths as well. The relaxing of safer sex practices so greatly enhanced their sex life that they decided, for the foreseeable future, not to expand their sexual repertoire to include sex with other people.

For gay men, feelings about anal penetration with and without a condom, drinking semen, sexual exclusivity, the specter of transmitting/contracting HIV and how each of these issues directly relate to trust, feeling emotionally safe, close, vulnerable and maintaining a rich shared erotic life has the potential either to dampen desire and intimacy or increase it. For some gay couples, condoms are a validation of their love and commitment to one another; for others, it is a barrier that prevents them from moving closer. For most couples, there is always some ambivalence about whatever sexual choices they are making. Therapy can provide what may be the only venue where both partners have the opportunity to discover and express the multiple meanings as well as feelings that arise in relation to these highly fraught issues.

COUNTERTRANSFERENCE ISSUES

Many therapists, gay or otherwise, have a challenging time with sexual practices that are frowned upon by the culture-at-large–anal sex, open relationships, "kinky" sex and group sex, etc. (Shernoff, 1988)–and are unlikely to be judgment-neutral about them. In the matter of preventing HIV and other STDs, however, a certain comfort level in discussing these topics is essential for effective therapeutic intervention. It is incumbent upon the therapist to create a treatment environment in which the patient feels safe enough to discuss any and all forms of sexual behavior; otherwise, discussion of the crucial issues of autonomy, (forbidden) desire, sexual self-confidence, and interpersonal intimacy will almost certainly be constrained from the onset, if not foreclosed.

Gay male therapists working with gay men face a particular challenge: it is all too easy for them to project their own feelings into discussions of safer sex issues. Every gay male therapist, regardless of his HIV status, has had to decide how he was going to handle these issues in his own life. Glassman, and Frederick (1998) describe learning how to manage their ambivalence and anxiety about adhering to safer sex guidelines while facilitating time-limited therapy groups for HIV-negative gay men. Cheuvront (2002) contends that "blind spots in treatment are a danger which can arise based on preconceived notions and stereotypes of the HIV risk-taker" (p. 11). Listening to individuals describe behaviors that can spread HIV increases the difficulty of maintaining therapeutic neutrality. Many individuals judge themselves for having unsafe sex. It is understandable that therapists may also have critical judgments of individuals who are having high-risk sex. This is likely to occur, especially, if an HIV-positive individual does not acknowledge anything wrong with behaving in ways that can infect others. In such cases, therapists must be prepared to put any of their own emotional reactions in perspective to avoid their interfering in the clinical work with the patient. To achieve such a perspective, even seasoned therapists should consider either personal therapy, or private or peer supervision.

It is reductionistic to either pathologize sexual risk-takers as self-destructive, suicidal, damaged individuals or to believe that "for some gay men danger is a permanent fetish" (Savage, 1999, p. 62). Cheuvront (2002) correctly notes that "the meanings of sexual risk-taking are as varied as our patients" and that simplistic explanations and understandings can "assuage the clinician's anxiety by making that which is complex and subject to individual differences appear less mysterious and knowable. Yet, this is not a luxury that clinicians have" (p. 15). The therapist's task is to help individuals articulate the particular meanings of their high-risk behaviors. Forstein (2002) asks: "Can care for the soul and care for the psyche always occur in the context of caring for the body?" (p. 38). Cheuvront (2002) suggests that for many gay men, self-care may indeed include taking risks. Forstein (2002) adds that "the question becomes one of understanding the nature of the risk and whether that particular risky behavior alone can attend to the needs inherent in the behavior" (p. 42).

Sexual behaviors hold various meanings for individuals which can evolve over time. To help individuals assess the importance and nuances of specific sexual acts, Drescher (1998) discusses the concept of sexual hierarchies. Citing Schwartz (1995), he defines sexual hierarchies as "referring to the ordering of sexual practices as better or worse in terms of some implicit or explicit value system" (Drescher, p. 217). In therapy with individuals taking sexual risks, it is useful to ask explicitly about the person's sexual behaviors and the hierarchical meanings that each of the risky behaviors holds for the individual in terms of satisfying both their intrapsychic as well as interpersonal needs and desires.

To do this in an effective way, however, Drescher (1998) further notes that "the therapist must be aware of his or own value system, including the kind of sexual hierarchy to which he or she adheres as well as the extent to which the theory he or she has learned has embedded within it sexual hierarchical judgments" (p. 217). It is often "not an easy matter to disentangle these different kinds of value judgments from each other, especially when the patient himself is in conflict about his own sexual practices" (p. 217).

One dynamic that may contribute to a therapist's difficulty in empathizing with a patient who is having high-risk sex may be generational differences between the two of them. Blechner (2002) states: "Young gay men today may be lucky not to have lived through the terrible times of the early days of the AIDS epidemic, but consequently, many such people do not share the great sense of relief that the previous generation felt at being able to stay alive by mere condom use. Some instead feel resentment and deprivation at the constraints of safer sex" (p. 29). Blechner further suggests "it is easy for older people who have enjoyed condomless sex, yet survived the epidemic to be smug about how the tradeoff between condom use and safety is obviously worth it. For younger people, who in any case feel invincible, the subjective valuation of condoms, risk, health, and pleasure may be different" (p. 29).

CONCLUSION

Engaging in high-risk sex often is symptomatic of intrapsychic, interpersonal, or communal distress. When gay men have unsafe sex in response to depression, loneliness, isolation, a nihilist malaise, or in conjunction with the use of substances, treating the underlying condition is essential. Even when underlying conditions improve in response to psychotherapy and psychopharmacologic interventions, unsafe sexual behaviors may not diminish or cease. If therapists gauge clinical success solely on the basis of patients stopping unsafe sex, they are settig unrealistic goals for themselves and for their individuals. It is important to differentiate between not having safer sex and having sex that places the individual at risk for transmitting HIV. The therapist must help each individual evaluate whether he feels not having safer sex is adaptive for him, even if the therapist strongly differs with the position taken by the patient.[3] For example, as some of the above cases indicate, there are circumstances where not using condoms is completely nonpathological. " Men in mutually monogamous, HIV-negative concordant relationships are not at high risk for transmission of HIV if they only

have sex with each other–even if they have unprotected anal intercourse" (Hoff et al., 1997, p. 75). Therapists need to explore concerns
about trust, monogamy, and degrees of risk with couples contemplating
abandoning safer sex. Harm reduction is an especially useful and practi-
cal strategy in dealing with individuals who are wrestling with substance use and/or high-risk sex.

One therapeutic goal should be to facilitate individuals' talking about
what level of risk is acceptable for them. This involves helping individuals to evaluate their capacity for tolerating and managing uncertainty
and ambiguity, especially as this pertains to the potential for HIV
superinfection.[4]

Love is one of the most complicated factors motivating individuals
not to have safer sex. Lust can make people do some seemingly irrational things, but when it comes to irrational behavior, nothing compares
to love. For some people, love can be a healthy and empowering force.
For others, it is part of the intrapsychic and interpersonal mix resulting
in an unhealthy loss of autonomous sense of self. Many people, across
the spectrum of mental and emotional health, find that love is the orga-
nizing principle of their personality and self-concept. For these people,
sex and love become inextricably linked, and rather than risk losing
love they have unprotected sex. For people unable to differentiate between lust and love, unprotected sex often is an effort to hold on to the
illusion of, or the potential for, love.[5]

Psychiatrist Mark Epstein (2001) suggests that change results
neither from people getting rid of their problems, nor from their going into them more deeply. It comes from helping them to accept
what is true about themselves and working from there. He also proposes
that good psychotherapy consists of helping individuals to find their own
meaning in their lives as well in the interaction with the therapist, as opposed to being fed interpretations. These thoughts seem particularly relevant for therapists working with gay men around sexual decision-making
in the age of AIDS. The combination of sexual risk-taking, personal and
public health issues, self-actualization, desire, love, recklessness, self-
destructiveness, and self-expression on the part of patients can be vola-
tile. However, when these factors are mediated by the therapist's sense of
protectiveness, urgency, and concern for the individual's welfare as
well as a non-dogmatic ethics, the interface can be powerful. This
can make for psychotherapy sessions that are vibrantly alive, frus-
trating, challenging, and dynamic for both parties: a space of clinical
practice within which the art and skill of psychotherapy can meet and be
tested.

NOTES

1. The names of all individuals throughout this article have been changed to protect their confidentiality.

2. HIV "superinfection" is defined as a second infection with HIV, after a primary infection has been established. This is distinct from "co-infection" which is defined as the simultaneous transmission of two or more subtypes of HIV (Blackard, Cohen and Mayer, 2002).

3. An example of this is noted by Rofes (1996) and confirmed by my clinical observations when despite knowing the risks of certain sexual behaviors, some gay men consciously prefer to prioritize pleasure over possible longevity.

4. There is now evidence from three reports (Angel et al., 2000; Jost et al., 2002; Walker, 2002) that HIV superinfection can occur. Another study has shown that unprotected insertive anal sex and receptive oral sex with HIV-positive or unknown serostatus partners accounted for 15 percent of all reported sexual activity by seroconverters (Vittinghoff et al., 1999).

5. In discussing his attraction to the character of Camille, the late Charles Ludlam, principal founder of the Ridiculous Theatrical Company, described it as having "a lot to do with my feelings about love and the nature of love in one of its highest expressions. Is love, in fact, self-sacrifice," he asked, "or is there another way of expressing love?" (quoted in Kaufman, 2002, p. 138). Although he was not speaking about sexual risk-taking, the conundrum raised by Ludlam is one that therapists working with people who have unsafe or unprotected sex, even within a committed relationship, would do well to ponder.

REFERENCES

American Psychiatric Association (2002), *Diagnostic and Statistical Manual of Mental Disorders, 4th ed–Text Revision (DSM-IV-TR)*. Washington, DC: American Psychiatric Press.

Angel, S., Kravcik, E., Balaskas, P., Yen, A.D., Badley, D. Cameron, W. & Hu, Y.W. (2000, February), *Documentation of HIV-1 Superinfection and Acceleration of Disease Progression*. Paper presented at The 7th Conference on Retroviruses and Opportunistic Infections, San Francisco, CA.

Blackard, J.T., Cohen, D.E. & Mayer, K.H. (2002), Human immunodeficiency virus superinfection and recombination: Current state of knowledge and potential clinical consequences. *Clinical Infectious Diseases*, 34:1108-1114.

Blechner, M.J. (2002), Intimacy, pleasure, risk and safety: Commentary on Cheuvront's "High-risk sexual behavior in the treatment of HIV-negative patients." *J. Gay & Lesbian Psychotherapy*, 6(3):27-34.

Chesney, M., Barrett, D. & Stall, R.D. (1998), Histories of substance use and risk behavior: Precursors to HIV seroconversion in homosexual men. *American J. Public Health*, 88:113-6.

Cheuvront, J.P. (2002). High-risk sexual behavior in the treatment of HIV-negative patients. *J. Gay & Lesbian Psychotherapy*, 6(3):7-26.

Colfax, G.N., Mansergh, G., Guzman, R., Vittinghoff, E., Marks, G., Rader, M. & Buchbinder, S. (2001), Drug use and sexual risk behavior among gay and bisexual men who attend circuit parties: A venue-based comparison. *J. Acquired Immune Deficiency Syndrome*, 28:373-379.

Drescher, J. (1998), *Psychoanalytic Therapy & The Gay Man*. Hillsdale, NJ: The Analytic Press.

Elford, J., Bolding, G. & Sherr, L. (2001), Seeking sex on the Internet and sexual risk behavior among gay men using London gyms. *AIDS*, 15:1409-1415.

Epstein, M. (2001), *Going on Being: Buddhism and the Way of Change . . . A Positive Psychology for the West*. New York: Broadway Books.

Forstein, M. (2002), Commentary on Cheuvront's "High-risk sexual behavior in the treatment of HIV-negative patients." *J. Gay & Lesbian Psychotherapy*, 6(3):35-44.

Fries, S. (1998), A place where no one knows your name. *The Advocate*, 752:24-31.

Germain, C.B. (1981), The ecological approach to people-environment transactions. *Social Casework*, 62:323-331.

Gitterman, A. & Germain, C.B. (1980), *The Life Model of Social Work Practice*. New York: Columbia University Press.

Glassman, N.S. & Frederick, R. (1998), When seronegative gay male therapists work with seronegative gay male patients: Countertransference issues in time limited group psychotherapy. In: *The HIV-Negative Gay Man: Developing Strategies for Survival and Emotional Well-Being*, ed. S. Ball. Binghamton, NY: Harrington Park Press, pp. 43-60.

Guss, J.R. (2000). Sex like you can't even imagine: "Crystal," crack and gay men. *J. Gay & Lesbian Psychotherapy*, 3(3/4) 105-122. Reprinted in: *Addictions in the Gay and Lesbian Community*, eds. J.R. Guss, & J. Drescher. New York: The Haworth Press, pp. 105-122.

Halkitis, P.N. (2000). Masculinity in the Age of AIDS: HIV-Seropositive Gay Men and the "Buff Agenda." In: *Gay Masculinities*, ed. P. Nardi. Thousand Oaks, CA: Sage Publications, pp. 130-151.

Halkitis, P.N. & Parsons, J.T. (2002), Recreational drug use and HIV risk sexual behavior among men frequenting urban gay venues. *J. Gay & Lesbian Social Services*, 14:19-38.

Halkitis, P.N. & Parsons, J.T. (2003), Intentional unsafe sex (barebacking) among HIV seropositive gay men who seek sexual partners on the internet. *AIDS Care*, 15:367-378.

Halkitis, P.N., Parsons, J.T. & Wilton, L. (2003a), Barebacking, among gay and bisexual men in New York City. *Archives Sexual Behavior*, 32:351-358.

Halkitis, P.N., Parsons, J.T. & Wilton, L. (2003b), An exploratory study of contextual and situational factors related to methamphetamine use among gay and bisexual men in New York City. *J. Drug Issues*, 33:413-432.

Halkitis, P.N., Wilton, L., Parsons, J.T. & Hoff, C. (2004), Correlates of sexual risk-taking behavior among HIV seropositive gay men in seroconcordant primary partner relationships. *Psychology, Health, & Medicine*, 9: 99-113.

Hoff, C., Stall, R.D., Paul, J., Acree, M., Daigle, D., Phillips, K., Kegeles, S. et al. (1997), Differences in sexual behavior among HIV discordant and concordant gay men in primary relationships. *J. AIDS & Human Retrovirology*, 14:72-78.

Jost, S., Bernard, M.C., Kaiser, L., Yerly, S., Hirschel, S., Assia, S., Autran, B. et al. (2002), A patient with HIV-1 superinfection. *New England Journal Medicine*, 347:731-736.

Kaufman, D. (2002), *Ridiculous! The Theatrical Life and Times of Charles Ludlam*. New York: Applause Theater and Cinema Books.

Kelly, J.A., Hoffman, R.G. & Rompa, D. (1998), Protease inhibitor combination therapies and perceptions of gay men regarding AIDS severity and the need to maintain safer sex. *AIDS*, 12:91-95.

Kim, A., Kent, C. & McFarland, W. (2001), Cruising on the Internet highway. *J. Acquired Immune Deficiency Syndromes*, 28:89-93.

Kippax, S., Crawford, J., Davis, M., Rodden, P. & Dowsett, G. (1993), Sustaining safe sex: A longitudinal study of a sample of homosexual men. *AIDS*, 7:257-63.

Leigh, B.C. (1990), The relationship of substance used during sex to high-risk sexual behavior. *J. Sex Research*, 27:199-213.

Mattison, A.M., Ross, M.W., Wolfson, T., Franklin D. & the HIV Neurobehavioral Research Center (2001), Circuit party attendance, club drug use, and unsafe sex in gay men. *J. Substance Abuse*, 13:19-126.

McFarlane, M., Bull, S.S. & Rietmeijer, C.A. (2000), The Internet as a newly emerging risk environment for sexually transmitted diseases. *J. American Medical Association*, 284:443-446.

Osborne, D. (2002), A holistic approach to health: GMHC to fold multiple life issues with HIV prevention. *Gay City*, 1:10, Oct 11-17.

Prestage, G., Kippax, S., Noble, J., Crawford, D. & Baxter, D. (1994). Sydney men and sexual health: Negotiated safety in a cohort of homosexually active men. Annual Conference Australian Society of HIV Medicine, (Unnumbered abstract). 6:125, Nov. 3-6.

Remien, R.H. (1997), Couples of mixed HIV status: Challenges and strategies for intervention with couples. In: *Psychotherapy and AIDS*, ed. L. Wicks. Washington, DC: Taylor & Francis, pp. 165-177.

Remien, R.H., Carballo-Diéguez, A. & Wagner, G. (1995), Intimacy and sexual risk behavior among serodiscordant male couples. *AIDS Care*, 7:429-438.

Remien, R.H. & Smith, R.A. (2000), HIV prevention in the era of HAART: Implications for providers. *The AIDS Reader*, 10:247-251.

Remien, R.H. & Stirratt, M.A. (2002), At a turning point? HIV prevention among men who have sex with men. *Five Borough AIDS Mental Health Alliance*, 4:1-10.

Remien, R.H., Wagner, G, Dolezal, C. & Carballo-Diéguez, A. (2001), Factors associated with HIV sexual risk behavior in male couples of mixed HIV status. *J. Psychology & Human Sexuality*, 13:31-48.

Rofes, E. (1996), *Reviving the Tribe: Regenerating Gay Men's Sexuality and Culture in the Ongoing Epidemic*. Binghamton, NY: Harrington Park Press.

Royce, R.A., Sena, A., Cates, Jr., W. & Cohen, M.S. (1997), Current concepts: Sexual transmission of HIV. *New England Journal Medicine*, 336:1072-1079.

Savage, D. (1999), The thrill of living dangerously. *Out Magazine*, pp. 62, 64, 118, March.

Schwartz, D. (1995), Current psychoanalytic discourses on sexuality: Tripping over the body. In: *Disorienting Sexualities*, eds. T. Domenici & R.C. Lesser. New York: Routledge, pp. 115-126.

Shernoff, M. (1988), Integrating safer sex into social work practice. *Social Casework*, 69:334-339.

Shernoff, M. (2002), Body image, working out and therapy. *J. Gay & Lesbian Social Services*, 14:89-94.

Springer, E. (1991), Effective AIDS prevention with active drug users: The harm reduction model. In: *Counseling Chemically Dependent People with HIV Illness*, ed. M. Shernoff. Binghamton, NY: Harrington Park Press, pp. 141-158.

Stall, R.D. (2002), *Co-Occurring Psychosocial Health Problems Among Urban American Men Who Have Sex with Men Are Interacting to Increase Vulnerability to HIV Transmission*. Poster session, XIV International AIDS conference, Barcelona, Spain, July 7-12.

Stall, R.D. & Leigh, B. (1994), Understanding the relationship between drug or alcohol use and high-risk sexual activity for HIV transmission: Where do we go from here? *Addiction*, 89:131-4.

Stall, R.D., McKusick, L., Wiley, J., Coates, T.J. & Ostrow, D.G. (1986), Alcohol and drug use during sexual activity and compliance with safe sex guidelines for AIDS: The AIDS Behavioral Research Project. *Health Education Quarterly*, 13:359-371.

Stall, R.D., Paul, J.P., Barrett, D.C., Crosby, G.M. & Bein, E. (1991), An outcome evaluation to measure changes in sexual risk taking among gay men undergoing substance use disorder treatment. *J. Studies of Alcohol*, 60:837-845.

Vittinghoff, E., Douglas, J. & Judson, F. (1999), Per-contact risk of human immunodeficiency virus transmission between male sexual partners. *American J. Epidemiology*, 150:306-311.

Walker, B. (2002), *Harnessing the Immune System to Fight HIV Infection*. Poster session, XIV International AIDS Conference, Barcelona, Spain, July 7-12.

Index

BOOK ORDER FORM!

Order a copy of this book with this form or online at:
http://www.HaworthPress.com/store/product.asp?sku=5569

Barebacking

Psychosocial and Public Health Approaches

____ in softbound at $29.95 ISBN-13: 978-0-7890-2174-8 / ISBN-10: 0-7890-2174-9
____ in hardbound at $49.95 ISBN-13: 978-0-7890-2173-1 / ISBN-10: 0-7890-2173-0.

COST OF BOOKS _____

POSTAGE & HANDLING _____
US: $4.00 for first book & $1.50
for each additional book
Outside US: $5.00 for first book
& $2.00 for each additional book.

SUBTOTAL _____

In Canada: add 7% GST. _____

STATE TAX _____
CA, IL, IN, MN, NJ, NY, OH, PA & SD residents
please add appropriate local sales tax.

FINAL TOTAL _____

If paying in Canadian funds, convert
using the current exchange rate,
UNESCO coupons welcome.

❏ BILL ME LATER:
Bill-me option is good on US/Canada/
Mexico orders only; not good to jobbers,
wholesalers, or subscription agencies.

❏ Signature _____

❏ Payment Enclosed: $ _____

❏ PLEASE CHARGE TO MY CREDIT CARD:
❏ Visa ❏ MasterCard ❏ AmEx ❏ Discover
❏ Diner's Club ❏ Eurocard ❏ JCB

Account # _____

Exp Date _____

Signature _____
(Prices in US dollars and subject to change without notice.)

PLEASE PRINT ALL INFORMATION OR ATTACH YOUR BUSINESS CARD

Name	
Address	
City	State/Province	Zip/Postal Code
Country	
Tel	Fax
E-Mail	

May we use your e-mail address for confirmations and other types of information? ❏ Yes ❏ No We appreciate receiving
your e-mail address. Haworth would like to e-mail special discount offers to you, as a preferred customer.
We will never share, rent, or exchange your e-mail address. We regard such actions as an invasion of your privacy.

Order from your **local bookstore** or directly from
The Haworth Press, Inc. 10 Alice Street, Binghamton, New York 13904-1580 • USA
Call our toll-free number (1-800-429-6784) / Outside US/Canada: (607) 722-5857
Fax: 1-800-895-0582 / Outside US/Canada: (607) 771-0012
E-mail your order to us: orders@HaworthPress.com

For orders outside US and Canada, you may wish to order through your local
sales representative, distributor, or bookseller.
For information, see http://HaworthPress.com/distributors

(Discounts are available for individual orders in US and Canada only, not booksellers/distributors.)

Please photocopy this form for your personal use.
www.HaworthPress.com

BOF05